Patrick Cameron
DRESSING LONG HAIR

Patrick Cameron and Jacki Wadeson

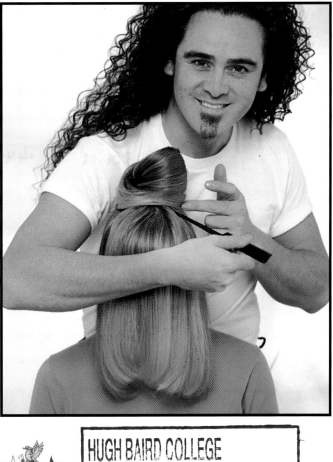

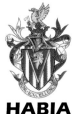

HABIA
Hairdressing And Beauty Industry Authority

THOMSON
™

Australia • Canada • Mexico • Singapore • Spain • United Kingdom • United States

ACKNOWLEDGEMENTS

Hair: Patrick Cameron.
Hair assistant: Marco Erbi.
Make-up: Debbie Findlay and Vanessa Haines.
Photography: Alistair Hughes.
Products: Wella Great Britain.
Equipment: heated styling appliances: BaByliss.
Equipment: brushes, combs, self-fixing rollers: Denman.
Accessories: Head Gardener, Knightsbridge, London; Alexandre de Paris.
Clothes stylist: Rachael Fanconi.
Clothes: Doyenne; Frank Usher; Freemans; Hyper, Hyper; Lara Jane; Looks Fashion; Influence; Marks & Spencer; Miss Selfridge; Next; Variations.
Bridal fashion stylist: Sue Allman of *Wedding & Home.*
Bridal dresses and accessories: Basia Zarzycka; Bridal Fashions (Brides International, Hilary Morgan, Mori Lee, Rena Koh); Dante (Ronald Joyce, London); Escapade; Leila Bejbordi; Linda Tidmarsh; Romantic of Devon.
Jewellery, head-dresses and veils: Adrien Mann; Elizabeth Edema; Hilary Morgan; Torq.
Flowers: Mulberry & Tomlinson, 11 Croxted Road, London.

With thanks to: Sue Callaghan; Annette Dennis; Jonathan S. King; Wilma Sladen; Liz Stovold.

THOMSON

For more information, contact Thomson, High Holborn House, 50-51 Bedford Row, London WC1R 4LR or visit us on the World Wide Web at: http://www.thomsonlearning.co.uk

British Library Cataloguing-in-Publication Data
A catalogue record for this book is available from the British Library

ISBN 1-86152-701-2

First edition published 1996 by Macmillan Press Ltd
Reprinted 2000 by Thomson Learning
Reprinted 2002 by Thomson

Printed in Italy by Canale

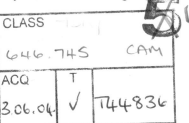

CONTENTS

FOREWORD

It never fails to amaze me that hairdressing produces many of the world's best entertainers, and Patrick Cameron without doubt is the most exciting personality in hairdressing today. On stage he reigns supreme from when the music starts. His brush action is delicate and precise and he ends with a flourish, a blast of hairspray and a perfect bow to the audience.

Patrick's dynamic style, attitude and creativity are captured in this book and today's hairdressers can make all the difference in their salons by learning the simple techniques he uses.

Alan Goldsbro
Chief Executive, Hairdressing Training Board

INTRODUCTION

*D*ressing long hair has always been surrounded by mystique. Our aim, in this instructional book, is to dispel the mystery and show how anyone can create a galaxy of beautiful upswept styles by following a few simple rules and working methodically and neatly.

Once you have mastered the basic techniques it is so simple to build upon your knowledge and personalise the looks to suit the hair type, texture or occasion. Add a curl here, a quiff there, tong hair into tendrils – you will be amazed at what you can do.

Practice builds confidence and you will very soon find that dressing long hair is easy and fun. This book is perfect for anyone who wants to master long hair. If you are training to be a hairdresser, you will find that the techniques covered fulfil the long hair criteria

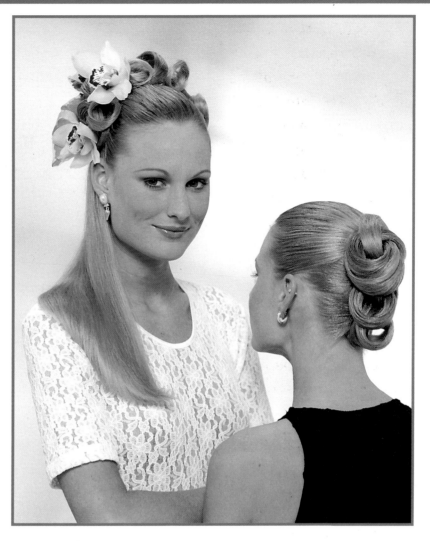

set out in NVQ Levels 2 and 3. If you are already qualified, the book will refresh your basic skills and give you the inspiration to take your work to new heights. Many styles are featured; all are simple, quick and very effective. As you work and create, remember Patrick's philosophy: less is always

more, and the simpler your styling the more beautiful the result.

Patrick Cameron
and Jacki Wadeson

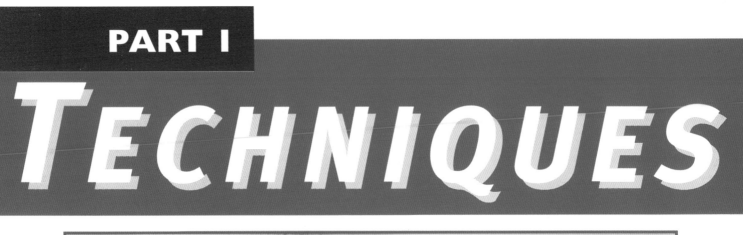

PART I

TECHNIQUES

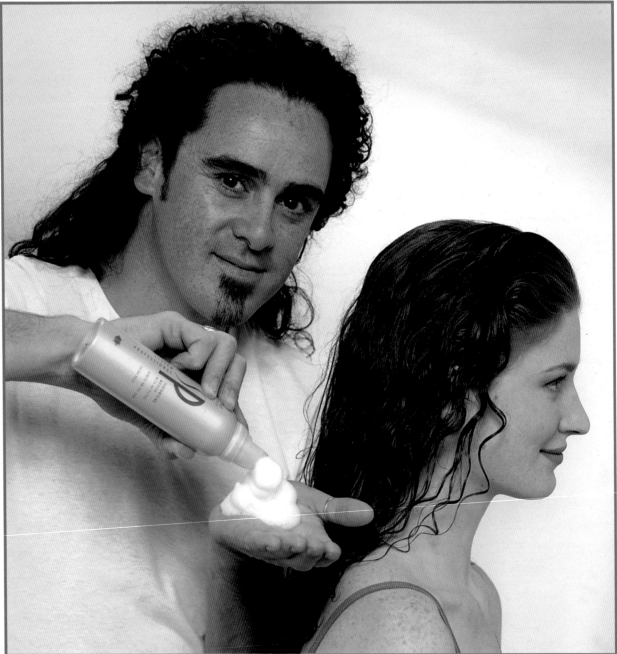

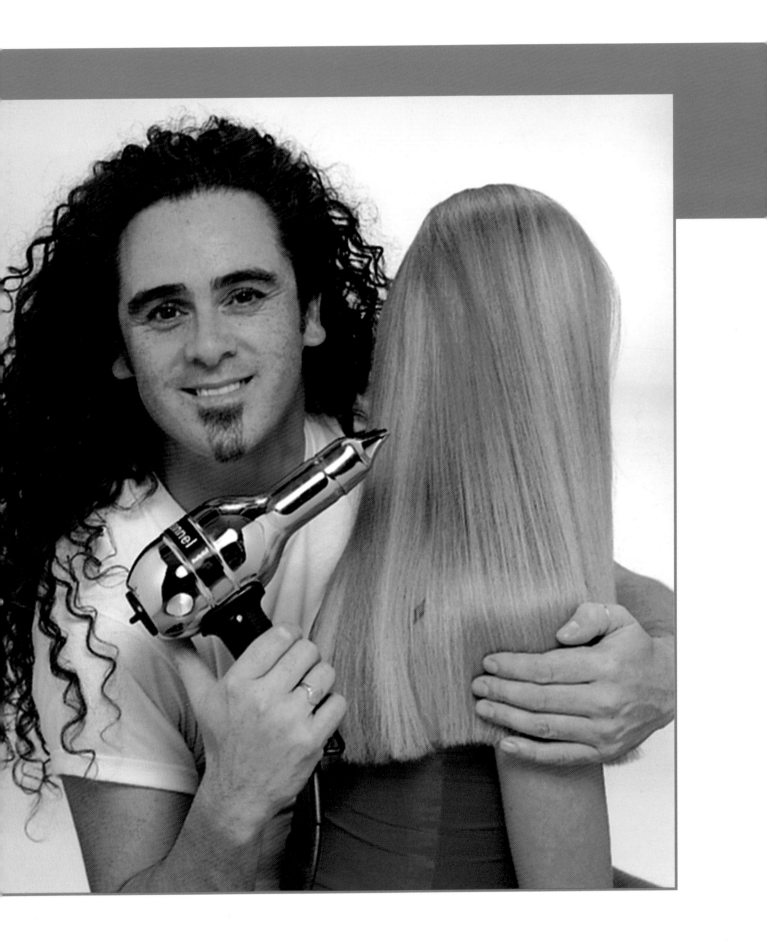

*A*s hair grows at the rate of 1.25 cm a month it means that long hair is several years old. It has borne the stress of physical and environmental assaults over a period of time and can easily become dull, dry, split and lack-lustre. To keep long hair beautiful it needs a care regime that begins with regular trims to remove any split ends and continues with the use of prescribed cleansers, conditioners and styling products specially designed for long hair.

*T*o strengthen, protect and add shine to long hair use specialist conditioning products.

A creamy conditioner is applied and massaged through lengths then left for 10 minutes to penetrate before rinsing.

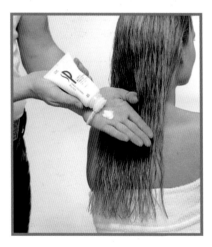

Strength and suppleness is increased with a protective spray.

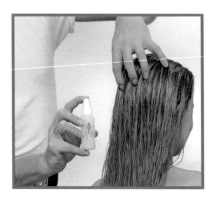

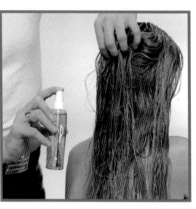

Specialist liquid repair products contain keratin and amino acids that penetrate deep into the hair shaft, filling in and rebuilding broken bonds. Use regularly on long hair to strengthen and form a protective seal that reduces the risk of future damage, making hair feel thicker and stronger.

*M*ousse is the most versatile styling product. Choose an alcohol-free version that contains conditioning agents and proteins to nurture and protect the hair.

Dispense mousse into palm of the hand – an amount the size of an orange is needed for long hair.

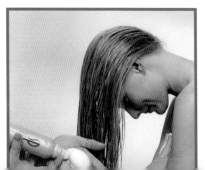

Work mousse through from roots to ends. It is important that the product is evenly distributed and essential that the root area is treated if you want to achieve maximum volume.

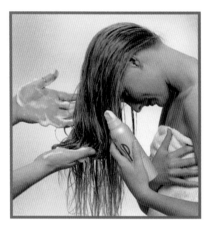

For bounce and movement, mist hair with a volumising spray. These sprays contain essential moisturisers that work to balance the hair's condition through its length. Good products give a natural hold with no hint of stickiness.

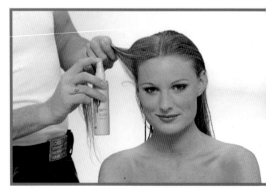

DRYING AND FINISHING

*P*rofessional heated styling appliances allow you to smooth, build body, straighten or curl hair efficiently and easily without risk of damage.

Blow-dry using a round bristle brush for smoothness. Use nozzle for direct air-flow and point dryer downwards to flatten cuticle and create maximum shine.

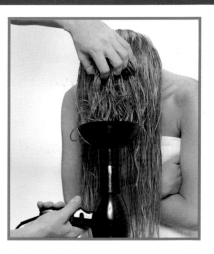

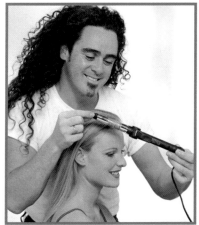

Diffuser-dry hair to encourage curl. First blot hair with a towel to remove excess moisture, then after applying a volumising spray or mousse allow lengths of hair to sit in diffuser cup. Lift hair with your fingers to ensure even distribution of warm air which increases curl formation.

Use tongs to curl tendrils of hair at sides. The thickness of the barrel determines whether you achieve small, medium or large curls.

Straighteners, which consist of two flat heated plates, can be used to iron out frizz or curl and give the smoothest possible finish.

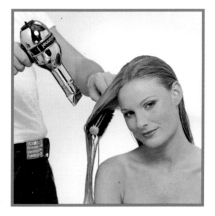

Add body using a vent brush which has a hollow centre that allows the air-flow from the dryer to pass through. The special pin patterns are designed to lift and disentangle even wet hair.

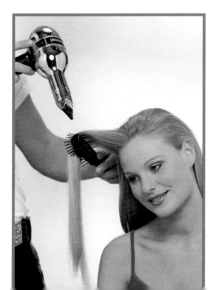

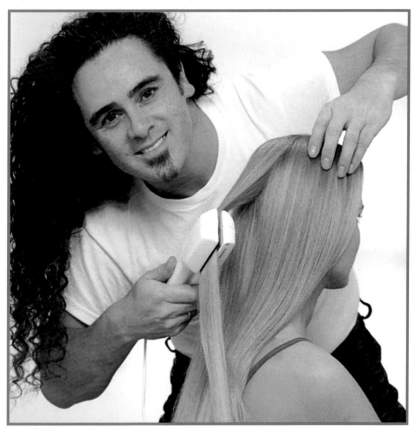

BASIC PONYTAIL

*U*se hat elastic to make your own hairbands which grip more securely and are kinder to hair than the conventional type which can sometimes tear or split the hair.

1. Cut a piece of elastic approximately 24 cm long.

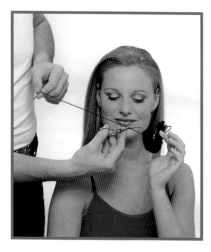

2. Tie into a circle and slip 2 hairgrips onto band.

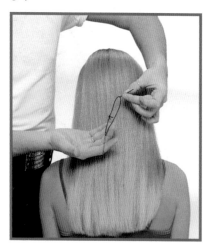

3. Hold ponytail in one hand and push one grip, flat to head, at base of where you want to secure hair.

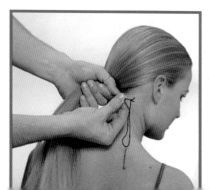

4. Pull elastic taut with the other hand and wrap tightly around ponytail, making sure elastic is wrapped over the top of the grip and not underneath.

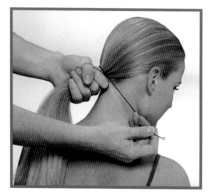

5. Continue wrapping until elastic will stretch no further.

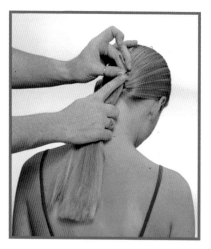

6. Now slide second grip up so you are just catching the elastic right at the end.

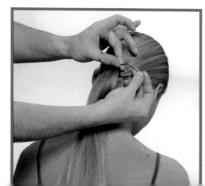

7. Push grip towards the scalp and under the hair to secure.

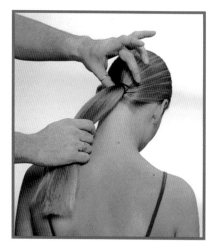

8. Completed ponytail.

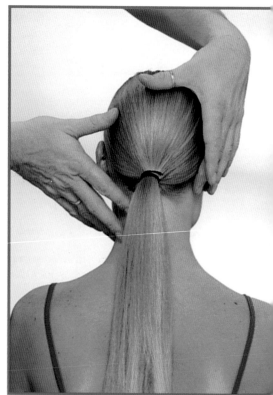

NETTING

Encasing sections of hair in fine hairnets makes long hair styling easier. Here's how to to do it...

1. Take a fine hairnet in a shade which matches hair colour.

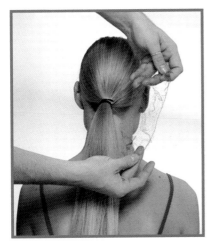

2. Hold one edge of hairnet taut over top of ponytail.

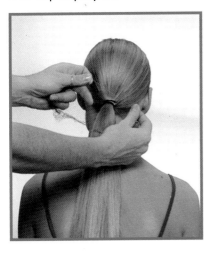

3. Hold ponytail up and wrap edges of hairnet round base of ponytail.

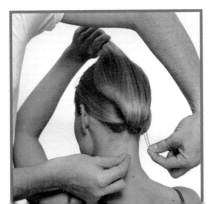

4. Secure hairnet at nape of neck using hairgrip to catch both sides of the net's elastic, then push hairgrip up and under the ponytail.

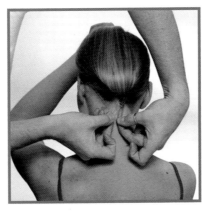

5. Shows hairnet attached to base of ponytail.

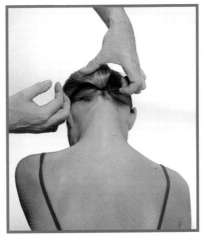

6. Allow ponytail to drop down and take hairnet over one hand.

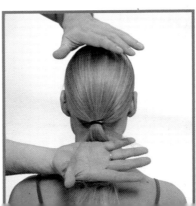

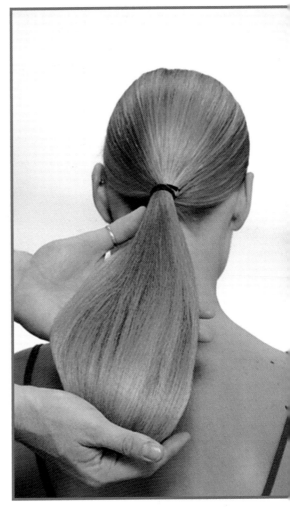

7. Encase hair in net.

11

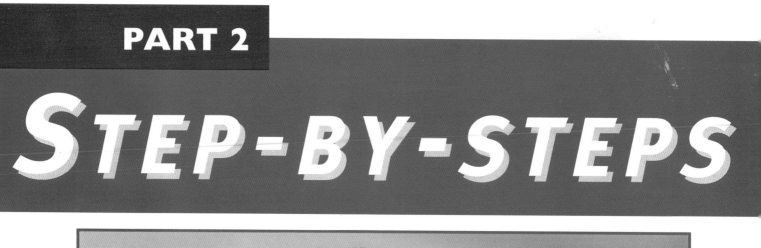

PART 2

STEP-BY-STEPS

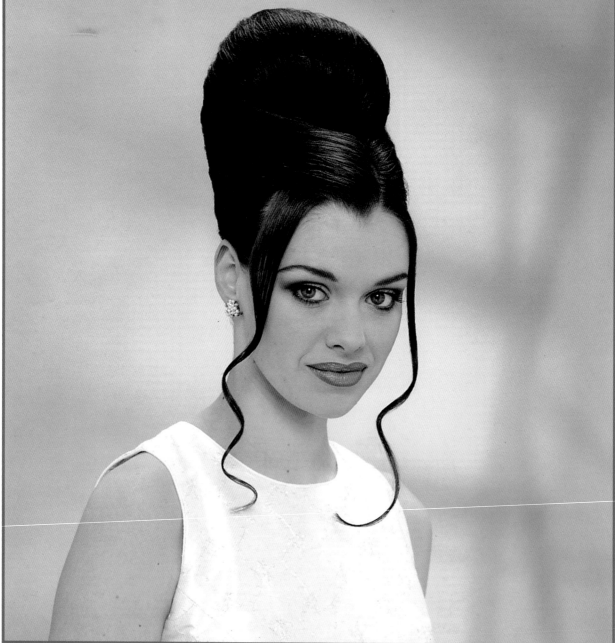

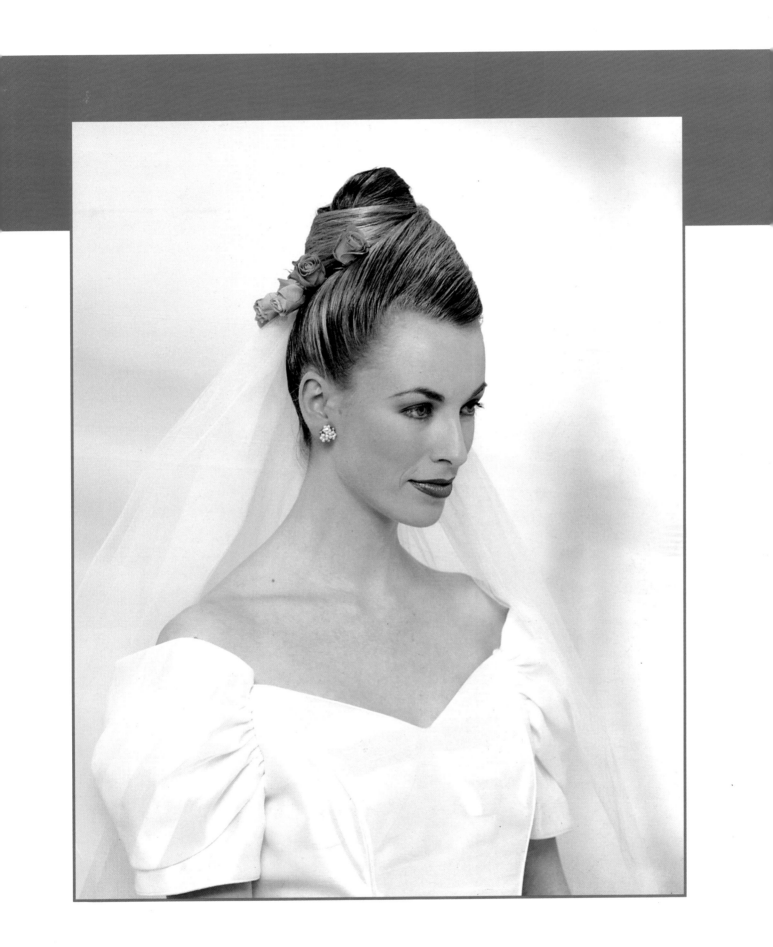

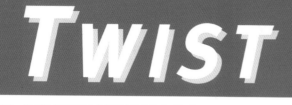

TWIST

Hair is simply coiled into a tight chignon.

Before

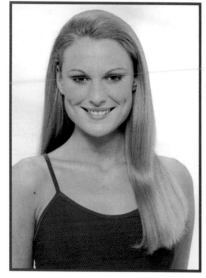

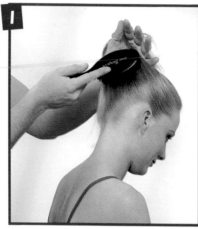

1. Brush hair up to crown.

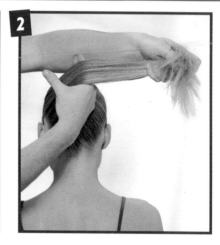

2. Clasp hair between thumb and fingers, holding ends with other hand.

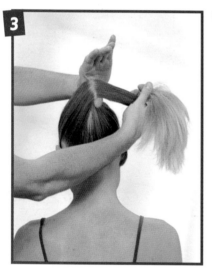

3. Pull hair ends taut over thumb.

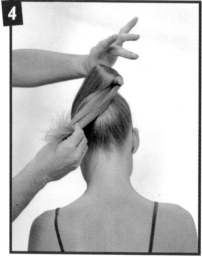

4. Twist hair under thumb and bring to other side, keeping the tension.

6. Push a hairgrip directly up seam of roll catching a little hair from underneath and from roll to ensure a firm hold.

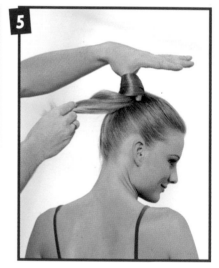

5. Place thumb on crown at a 90° angle and push roll of hair slightly forward.

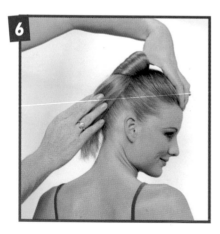

Tip
To get the smoothest possible finish, use a conditioning blow-dry lotion which maintains natural moisture and reduces static.

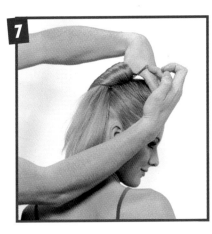

7. Repeat from top end of roll. You will only need three or four hairgrips.

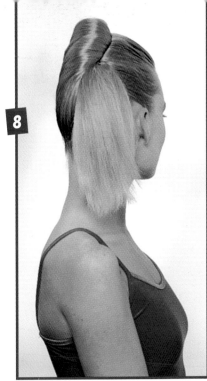

8. Shows first section completed.

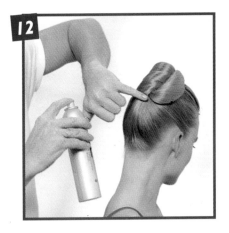

9. Smooth tail of hair round to front.

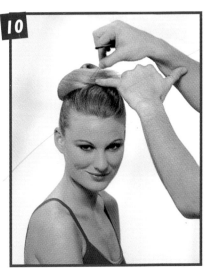

10. Secure at front with a hairpin.

12. Mist with hairspray.

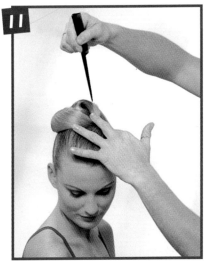

11. Use end of tailcomb to form hair into a curl and secure with a fine hairpin.

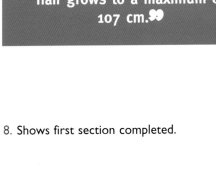

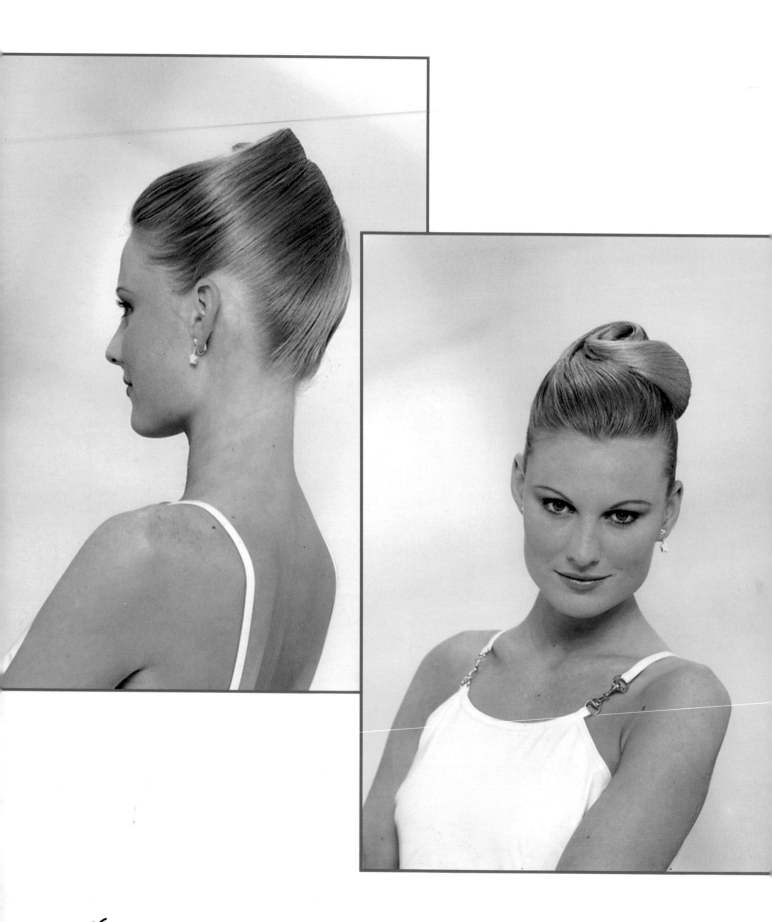

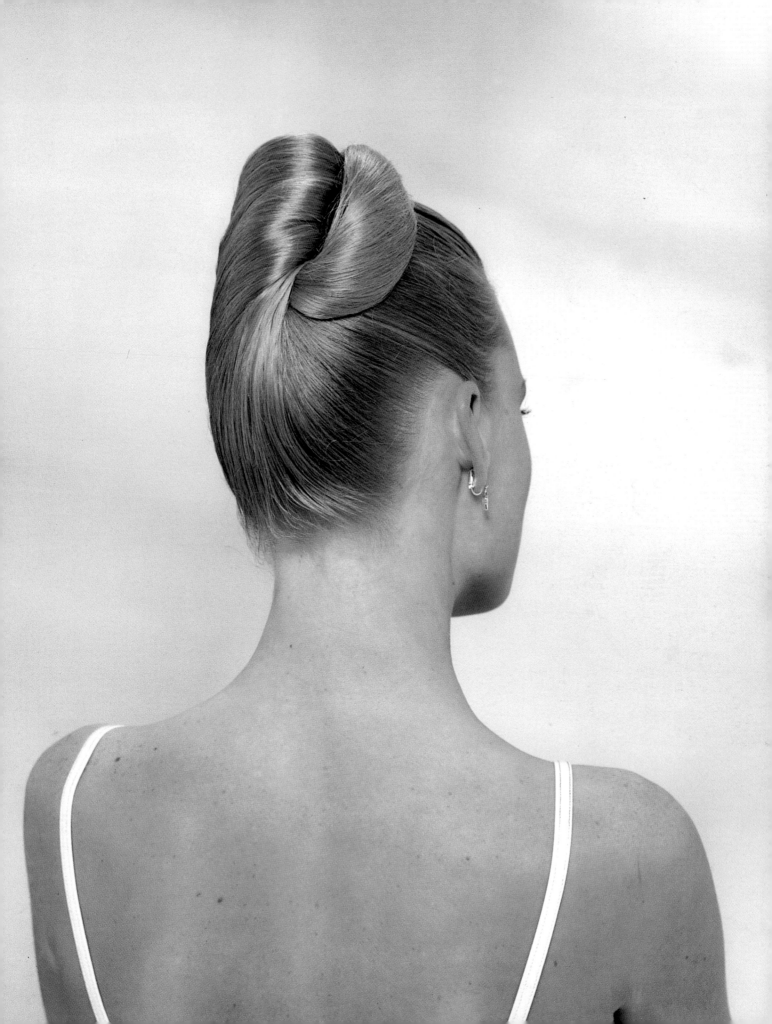

CASCADE

Natural curls are given texture, form and femininity.

Before

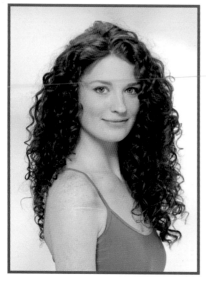

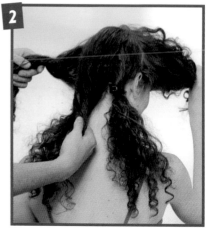

1. Divide off front hair from ear to ear.

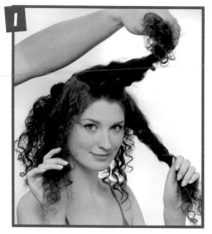

2. Divide back hair into three equal sections.

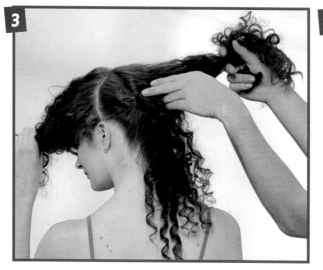

3. Secure each ponytail in a band, lifting each up 2–3 cm, as you fasten

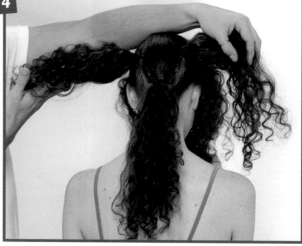

4. The three ponytails should form a triangle, the middle one being lower and quite close to nape of neck.

5. Take one ponytail and twist into a coil using a clockwise motion

6. Hair will begin to double back on itself.

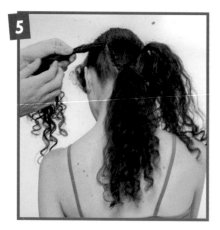

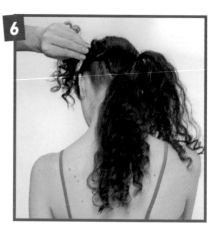

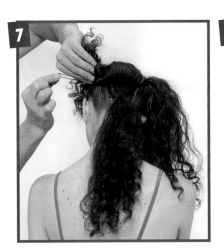

7. Secure with a pin and let ends fall. Repeat for other ponytails.

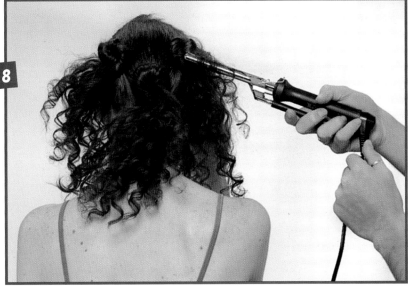

8. Redefine and smooth curls by tonging each one.

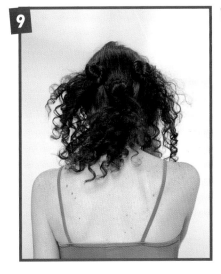

9. Shows tonged curls. Repeat for rest of back hair.

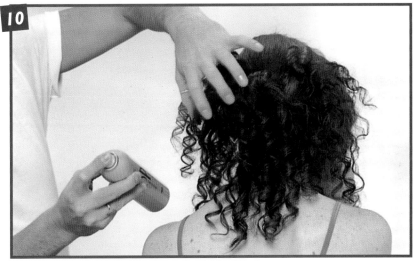

10. Mist with hairspray to hold re-formed curls.

Tip

Long, curly hair can look wild and unruly. By twisting into coils, weight is removed and hair looks more defined and elegant.

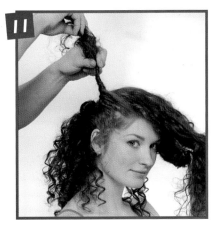

11. Section off one third of front hair and twist in a clockwise direction to form a coil as before.

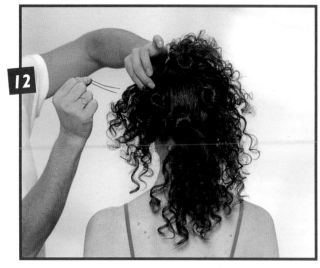

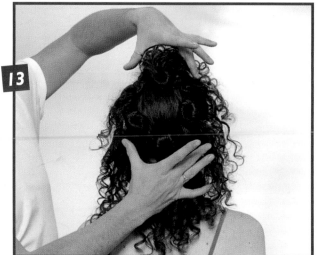

12. Repeat with other two sections and pin in place allowing tendrils of curls to fall.

13. Shows completed coils. Now arrange curls to create a halo effect.

14. Accessorise with pearl-tipped pins.

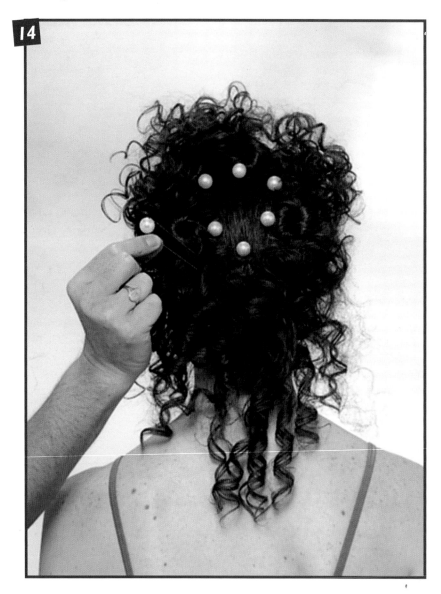

66 Markets, haberdashery departments of large stores and hair and beauty shops are all good hunting grounds for unusual hair accessories.99

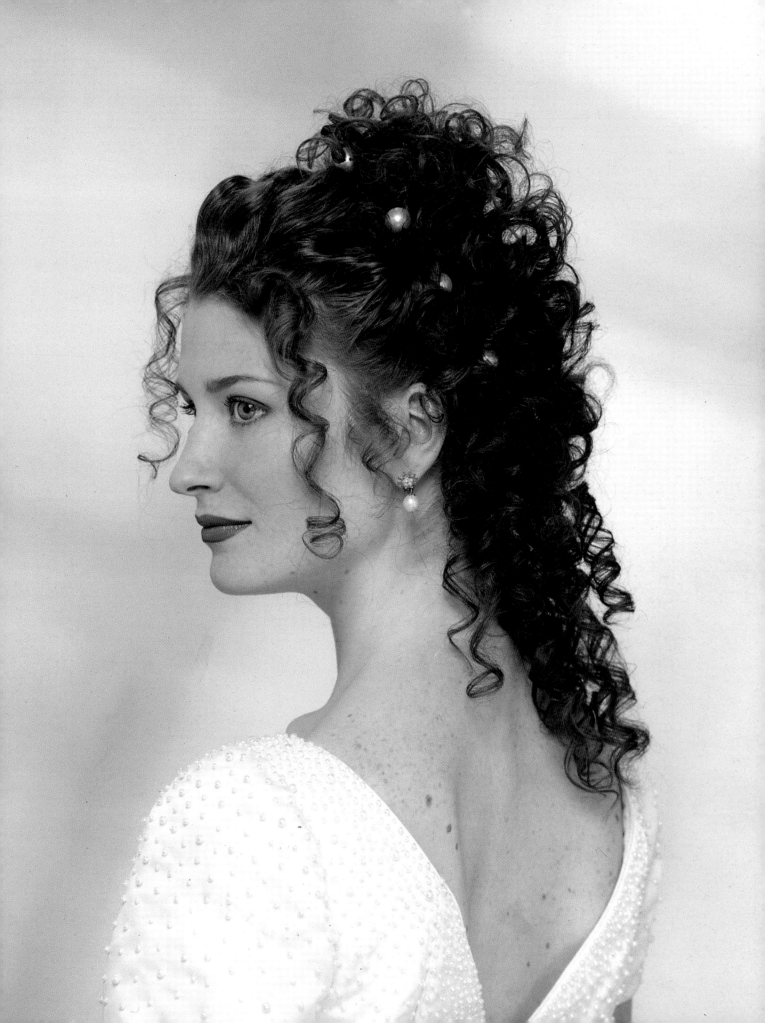

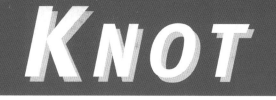

KNOT

Low chignon is created with a folding technique.

Before

 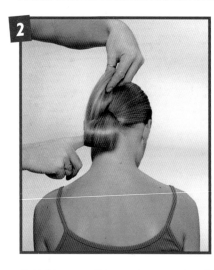

Tip

Wispy ends can be slicked into place by misting a little hairspray onto fingers and smoothing over hair.

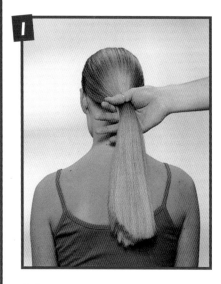

1. Smooth hair into a low ponytail.

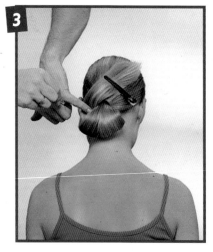

2. Fold ponytail into a large curl and hold in place with forefinger.

3. Bring end of ponytail up and secure with a section clip. Grip underneath.

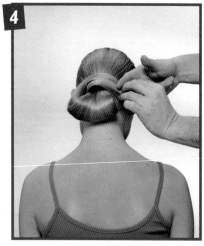

4. Wrap ends over and grip at other side. Mist with hairspray and add hair accessories.

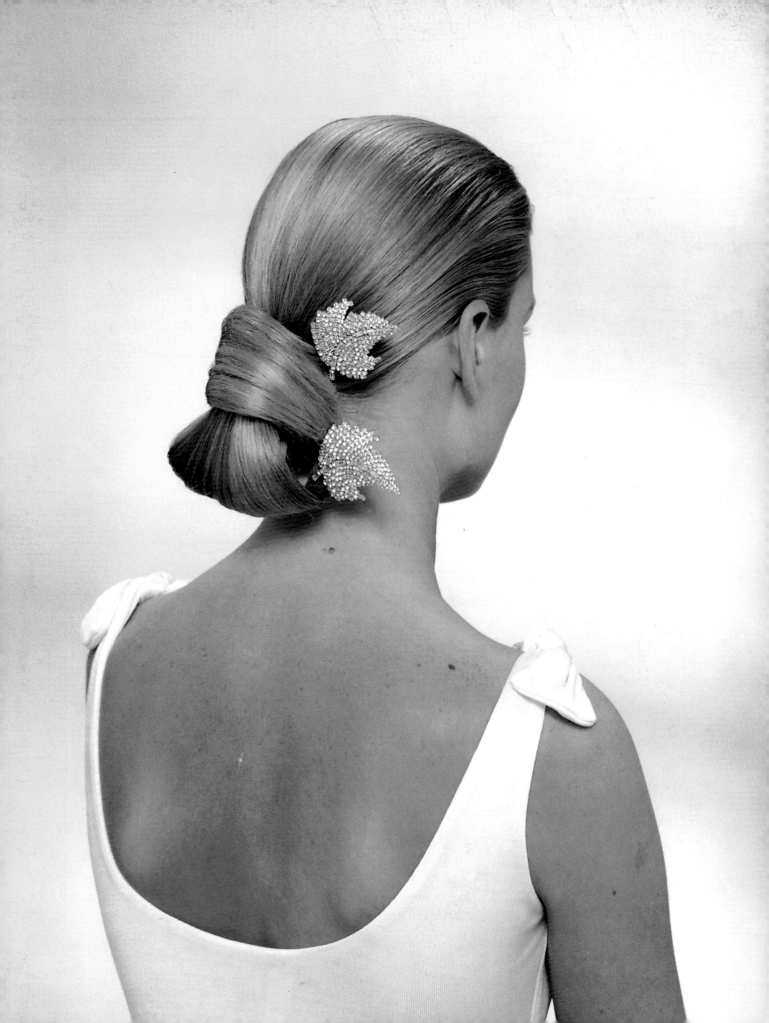

CLASSIC CHIGNON

Hair is twisted in a figure of eight.

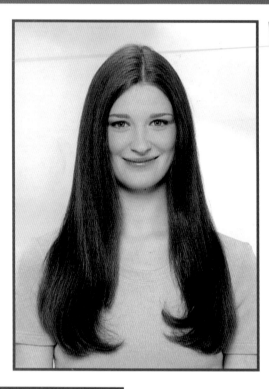

Before

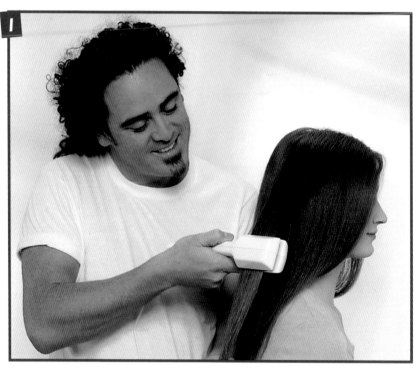

1. Straighten dry hair, a section at a time, using flat irons.

2. Reduce any hint of static by using a pure bristle brush to smooth hair.

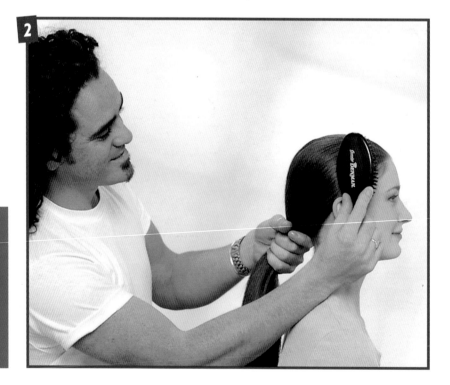

❝ Quills or pins in brushes can be made of bristle, plastic or nylon. The wider the spacing of the pins, the easier the brush will flow through the hair. ❞

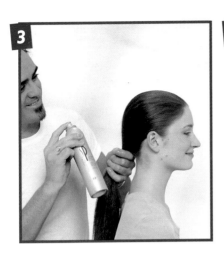

3. Mist with hairspray.

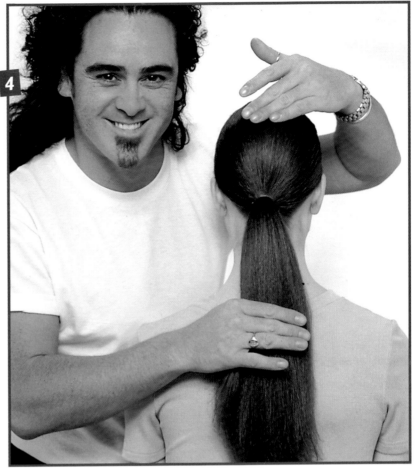

4. Secure hair in a low ponytail.

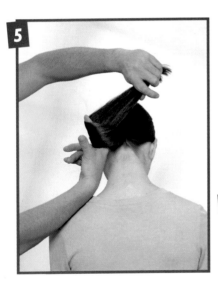

5. Twist hair round forefinger, holding ends of ponytail in other hand and taking tails over, not under.

6. Secure from top using a large hairgrip.

Tip

To make ponytail easier to handle, mist with hairspray and mould with hands before twisting hair.

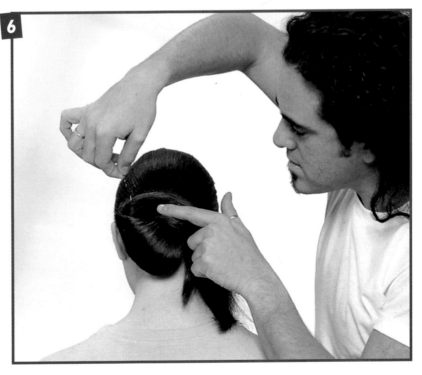

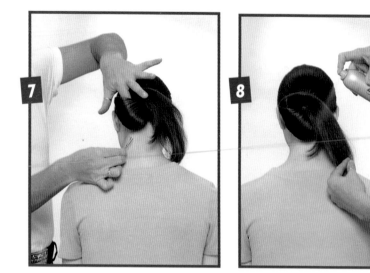

7. Repeat at base of pleat.

8. Mist tail with hairspray.

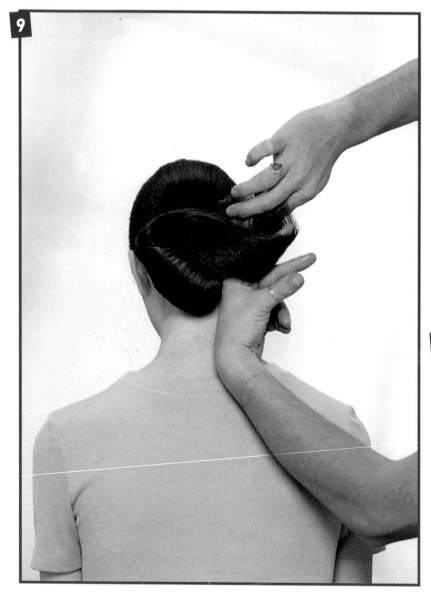

9. Twist tail round forefinger, curling in ends to form a figure of eight.

10. Secure with grips and add fresh flowers.

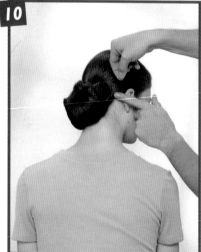

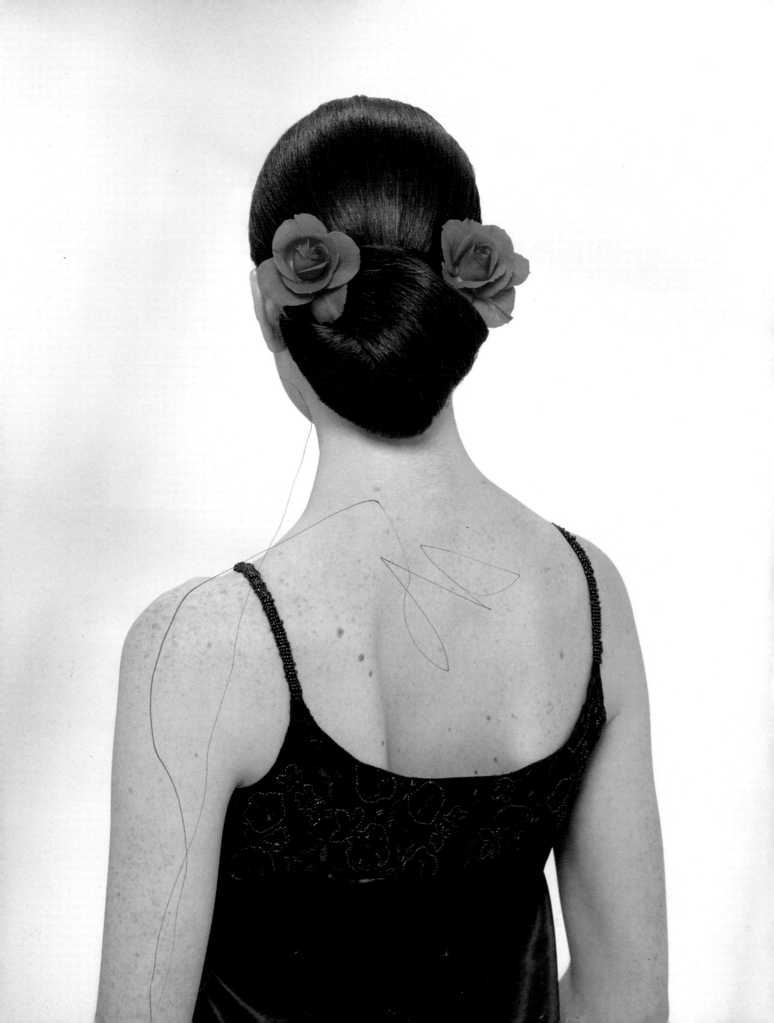

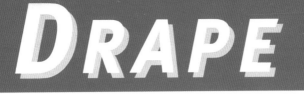

A topknot is given a sophisticated finish.

Before

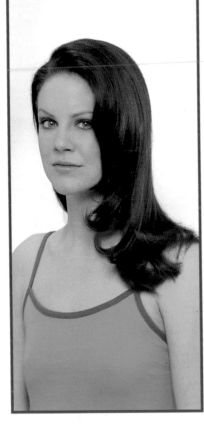

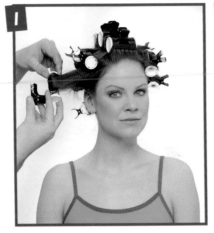

1. Foundation-set hair on heated rollers.

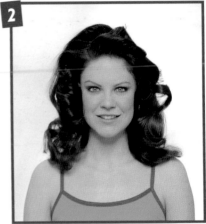

2. Remove rollers and run fingers through hair to loosen curl.

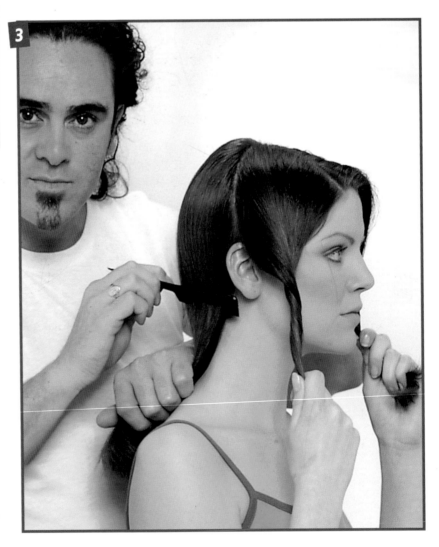

3. Part off back hair with a clean parting from ear to ear. Diagonally part front hair from crown to front hairline.

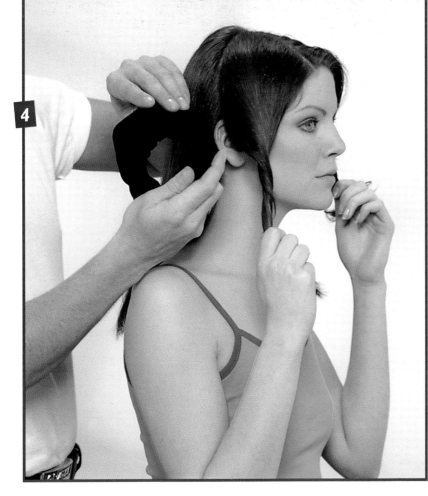

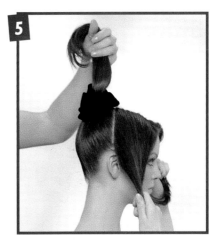

5. Use a bristle brush to smooth back hair upwards to crown, secure in fabric band.

4. Use a large fabric band that has some bulk as a 'bun ring'.

Tip

This is one of the simplest upswept styles and, with just a little practice, anyone can use this technique to put their hair up in minutes. For a professional finish it is important to brush the hair wide around the topknot.

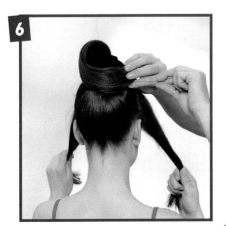

6. Swirl hair round fabric band and secure with pins.

7. Brush one side section, keeping it flat and wide as you sweep at a 45° angle towards crown before pinning in place.

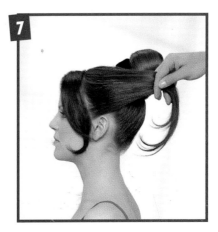

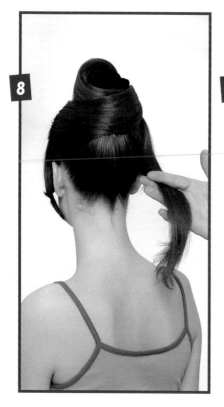

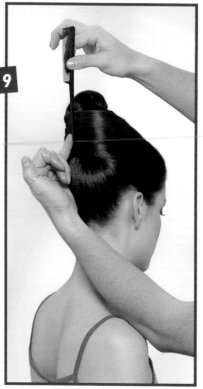

8. Take other side section, smooth and pin in same manner.

9. Use a tailcomb to tidy any stray ends.

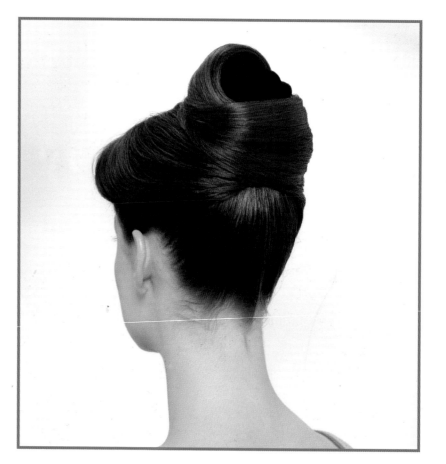

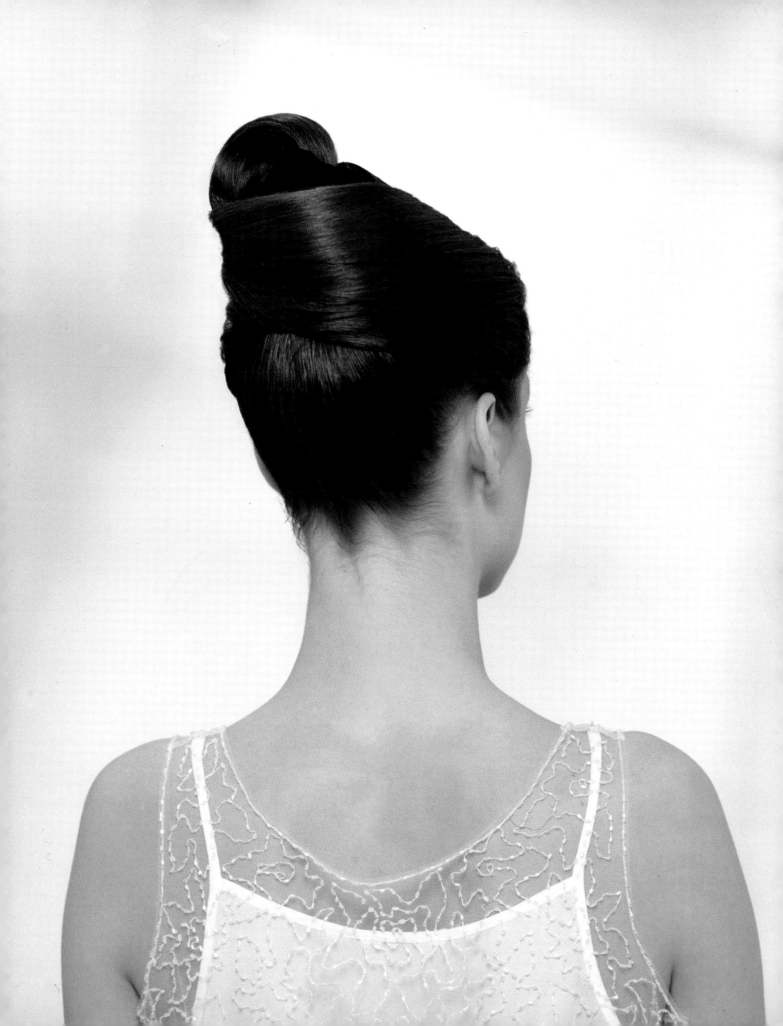

UNDER FLIP

Simply roll hair and knot for this classic look.

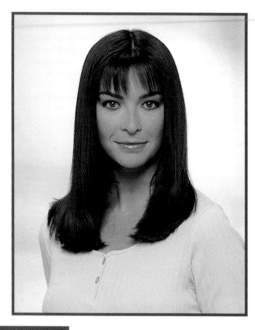

Before

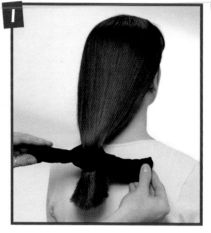

1. Brush hair smoothly back. Take a wired velvet band and tie in a knot approximately 8 cm from ends of hair.

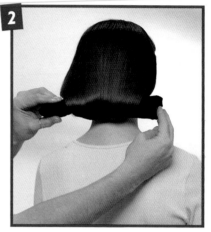

2. Roll velvet band under and up like a sausage.

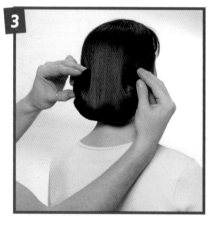

3. Twist ends of band together to secure before adding a pretty tiara of artificial or real flowers.

Tip

To get extra shine and reduce static, wrap a silk scarf round your hairbrush and stroke through hair.

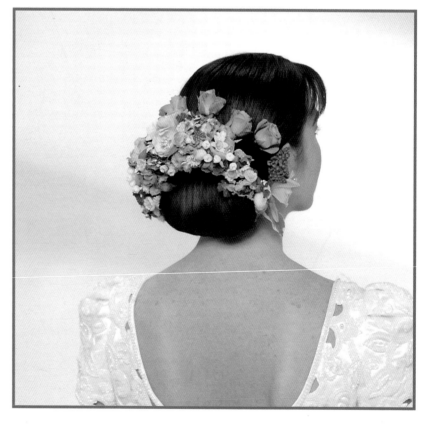

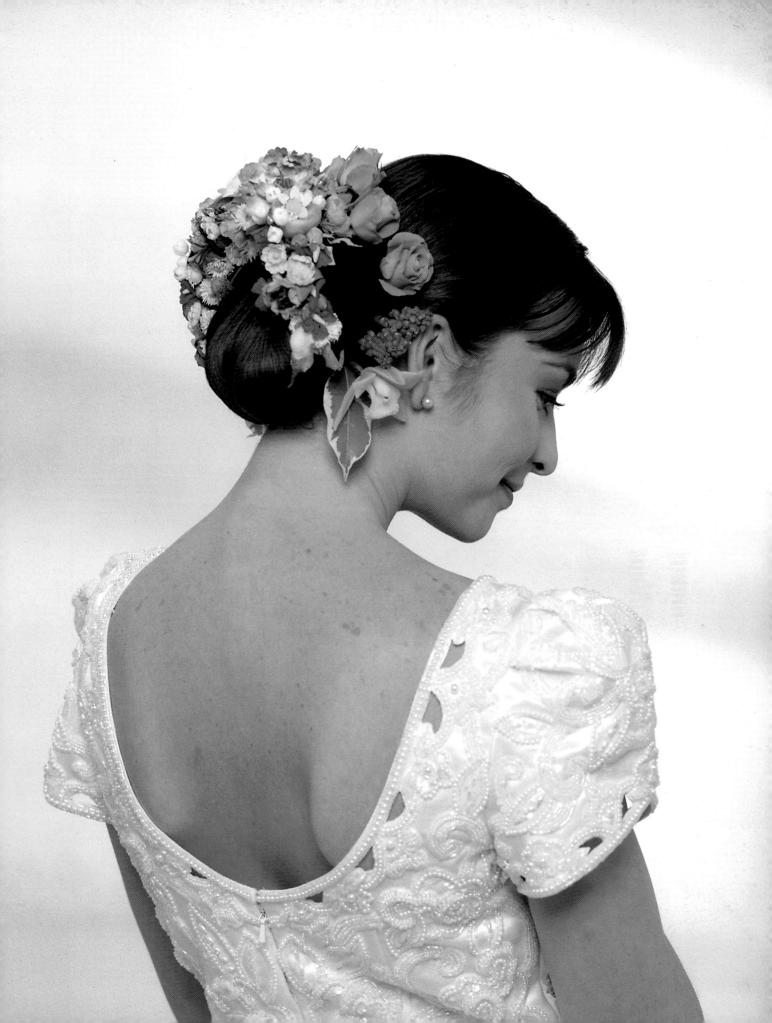

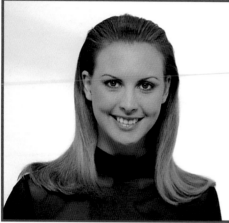

Before

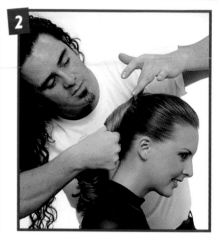

1. Using a bristle brush, smooth hair as if to make a ponytail.

2. From the pivot point of middle finger of your left hand, twist hair downwards with your right hand.

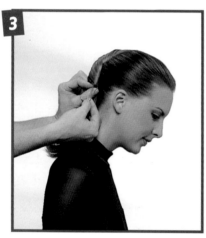

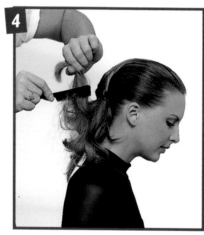

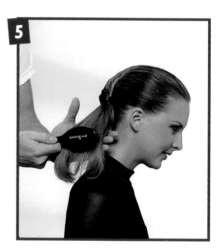

3. Grip in place.

4. Backcomb tail end.

5. Smooth top layer of tail hair.

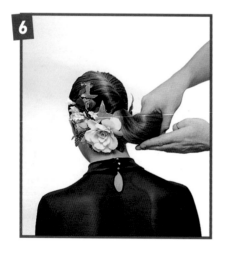

6. Pin one end of floral head-dress in place.

7. Curl tail of hair into a swirl and pin at top before pulling head-dress through centre and securing. Mist with hairspray.

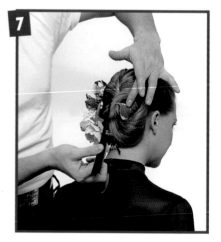

Tip

Use hairpins that match hair colour or try the invisible, non-reflective type.

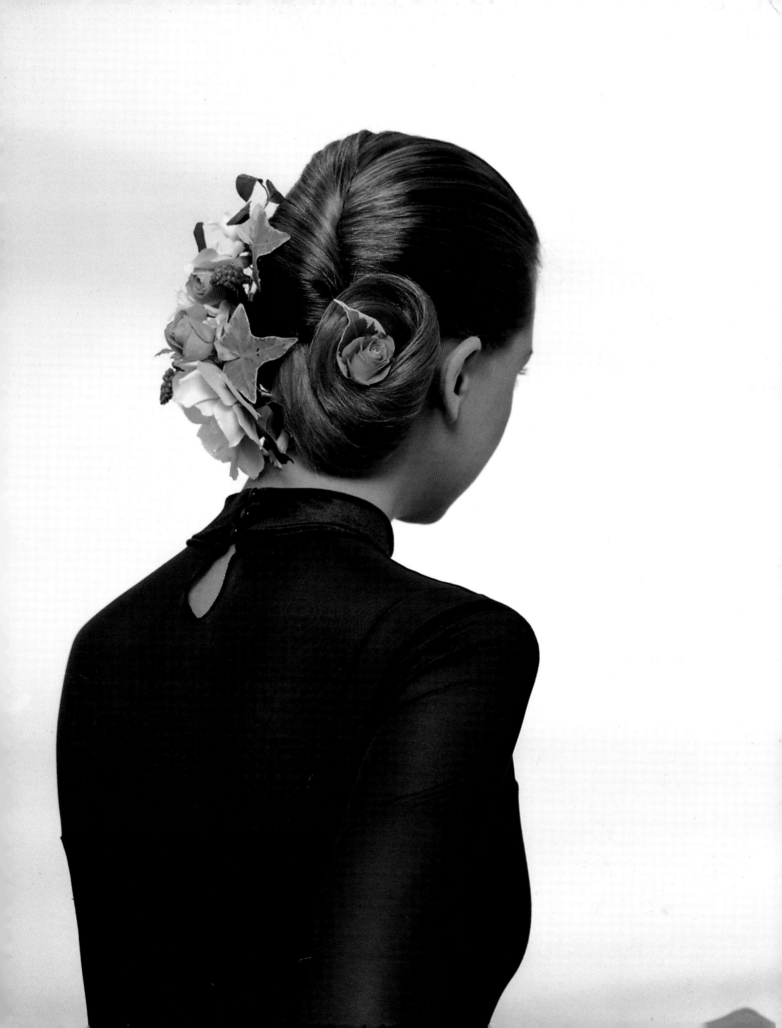

Before

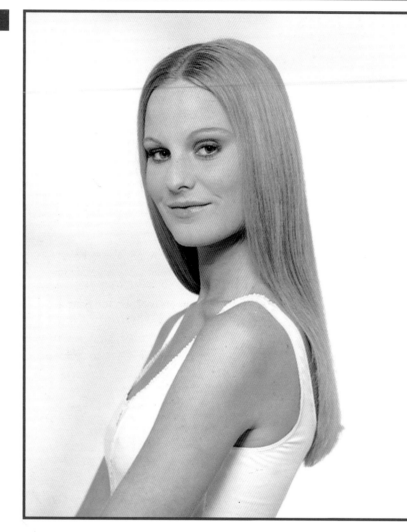

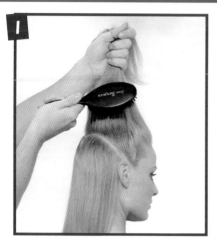

1. Section off top hair from ear to ear, and smooth over to front using a bristle brush.

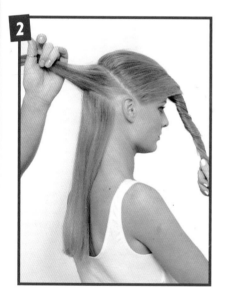

2. Take another parallel section 5 cm below the first and secure in a ponytail. Brush nape hair into a ponytail and secure in a band. Make sure that the hair from each ponytail overlaps each successive parting.

> **❝** Knots often occur on fine, dry hair, especially if it is split. Before brushing, use liquid restructuring conditioners that work by fortifying hair with proteins where needed. Gently disentangle with a wide-toothed comb, working from the roots up the hair shaft to prevent further damage. **❞**

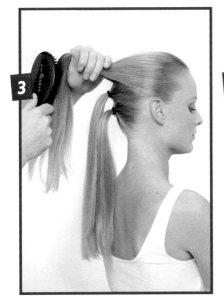

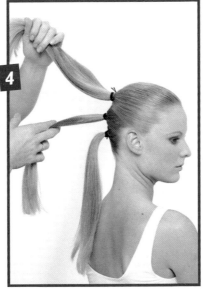

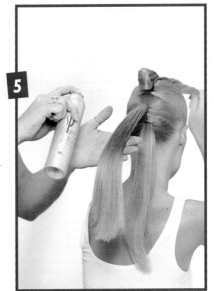

3. Take reserved front hair back and secure in a third ponytail. It is important to keep ponytails close together so each knot sits next to the other.

4. The ponytails should be aligned vertically.

5. Mist centre ponytail with spray and 'milk' hair with hands to dry spray and give the silkiest possible finish in preparation for tying a basic knot in the hair.

6. Coil centre ponytail to left, around forefinger.

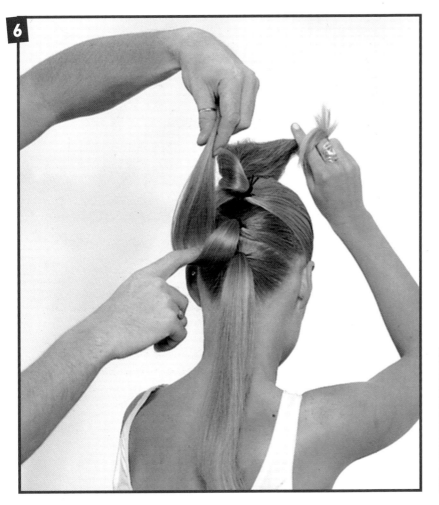

Tip
When misting sections of hair with spray, keep moving to get the finest possible coverage without undue wetness.

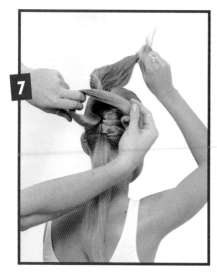

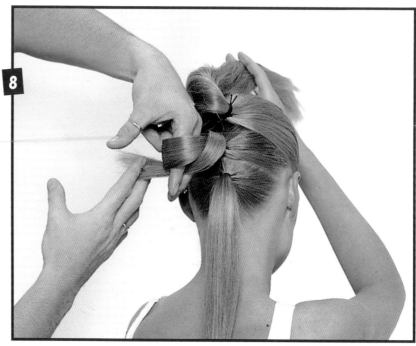

7. Pull tail end over to right.

8. Flip tail to left and up through centre of coiled hair.

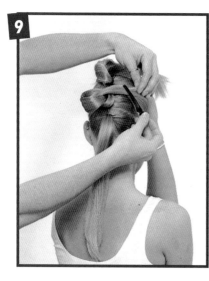

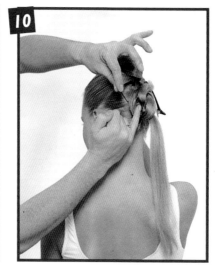

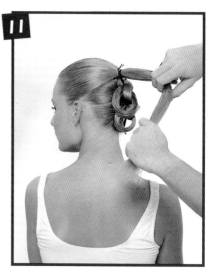

9. Secure end of tail with a section clip.

10. Use a hairgrip to secure coil.

11. Repeat same technique for lower and upper ponytails.

12. Secure tails to opposite side using section clips.

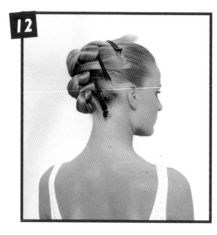

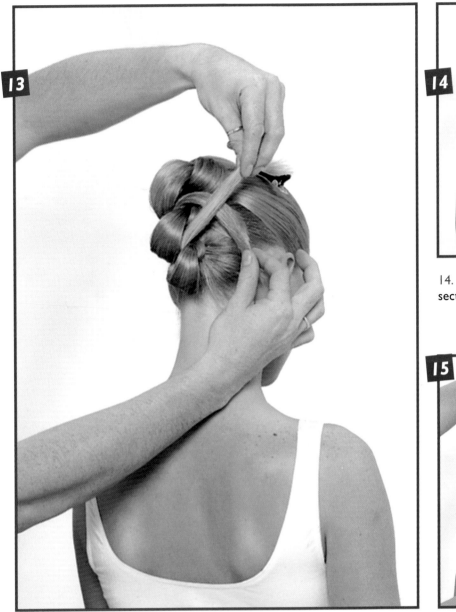

13. Now criss-cross lower tail with middle one making sure lower tail is on top.

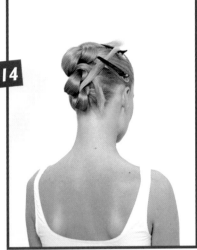

14. Secure the lower tail with a section clip.

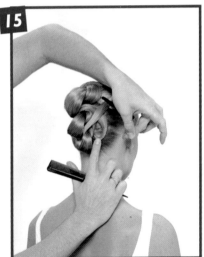

15. Pin curl the tail ends.

16. Repeat pin curl on middle tail and pin curl top tail to finish.

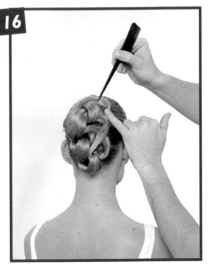

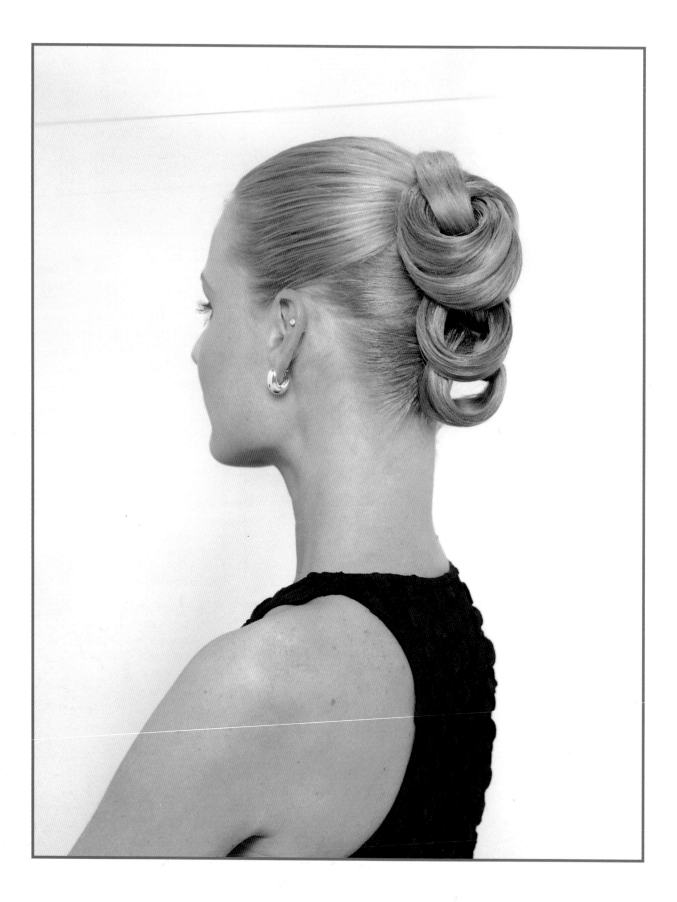

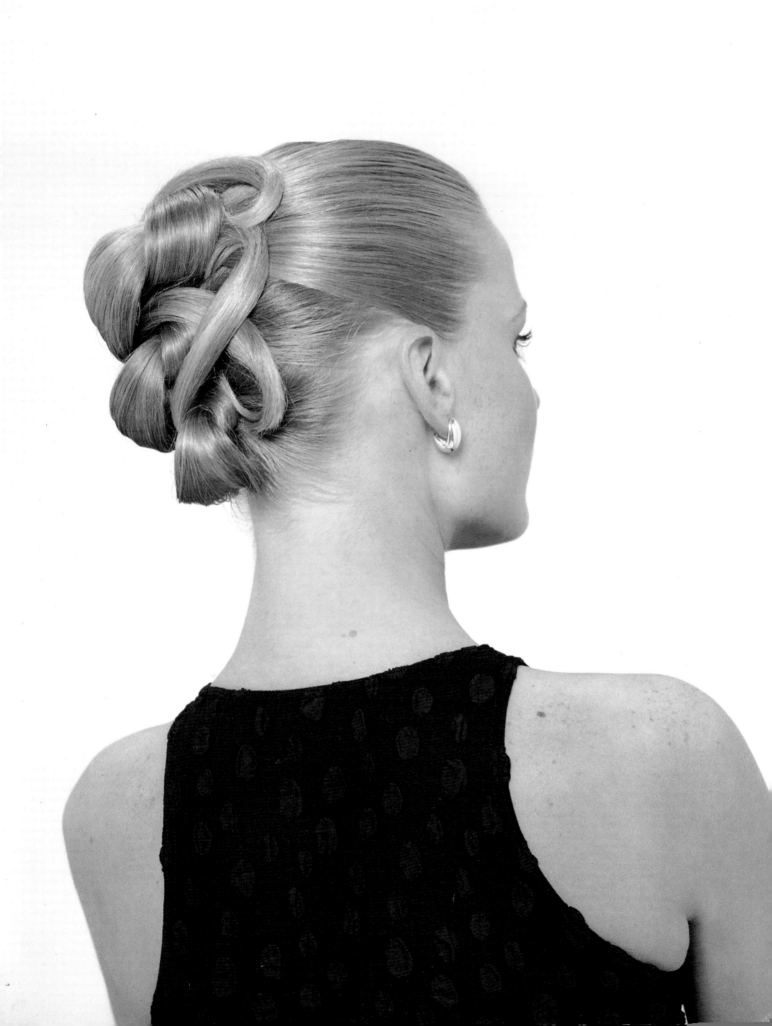

TWIRL

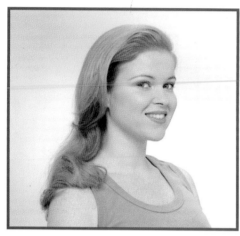

Before

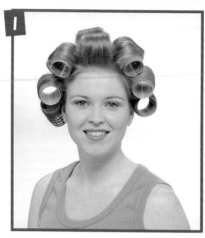

1. Mist dry hair with setting lotion and set on rollers.

❝ Rollers are the simple, easy way to create curls. Self-fixing rollers stay in place without the need for grips, pins or clips.❞

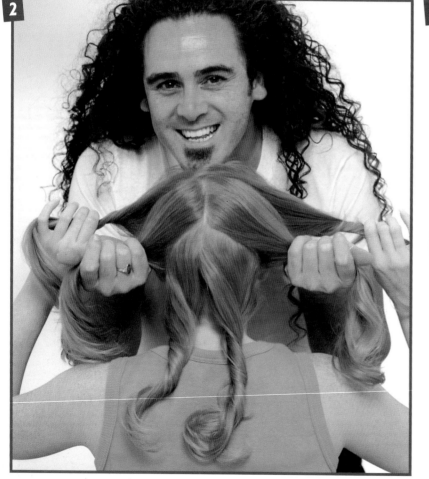

2. Remove rollers, brush hair and divide into six sections leaving front hair free. Twist each section to keep separate.

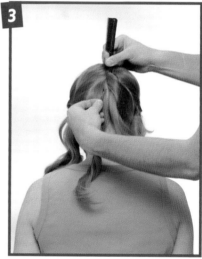

3. Twist one back section round and through in a figure of eight allowing tail to fall loose. Grip in place.

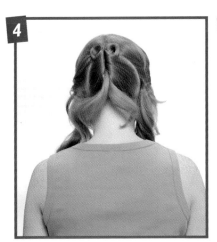

4. Repeat with other back section.

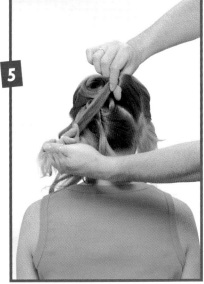

5. Take mid-side section, repeat figure of eight movement and pin.

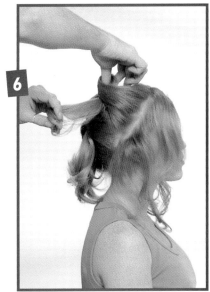

6. Take other mid-side section between thumb and forefinger.

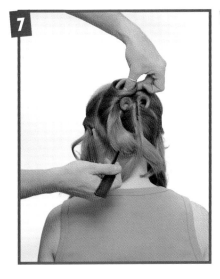

7. Twist in a figure of eight again and pin.

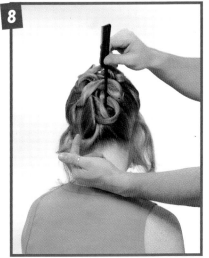

8. Shape tails of twisted hair into pincurls.

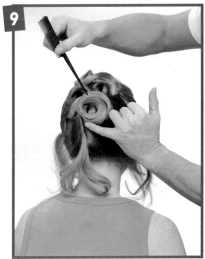

9. Continue twisting all tails into pincurls, pinning as you go.

Tip

To create maximum body when foundation-setting,
apply heat for 10 minutes, then allow hair to cool completely
before removing rollers.

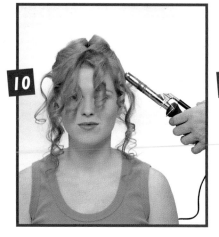

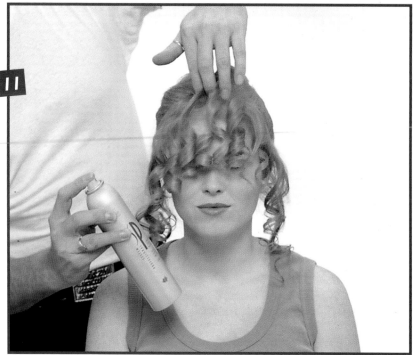

10. Tong front section of hair.

11. Mist with hairspray.

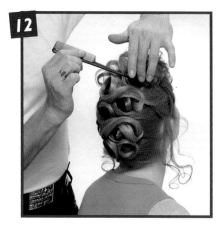

12. Carefully sweep back tonged curls, form into shape, arrange and pin as required.

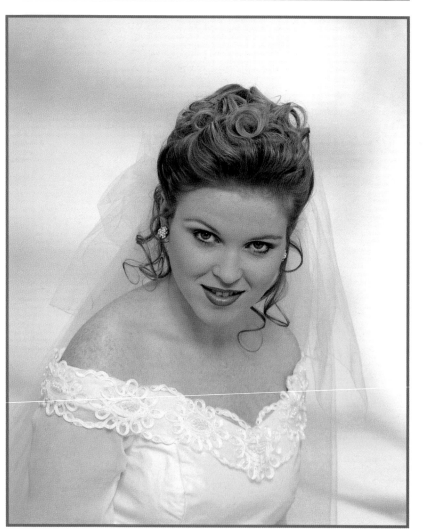

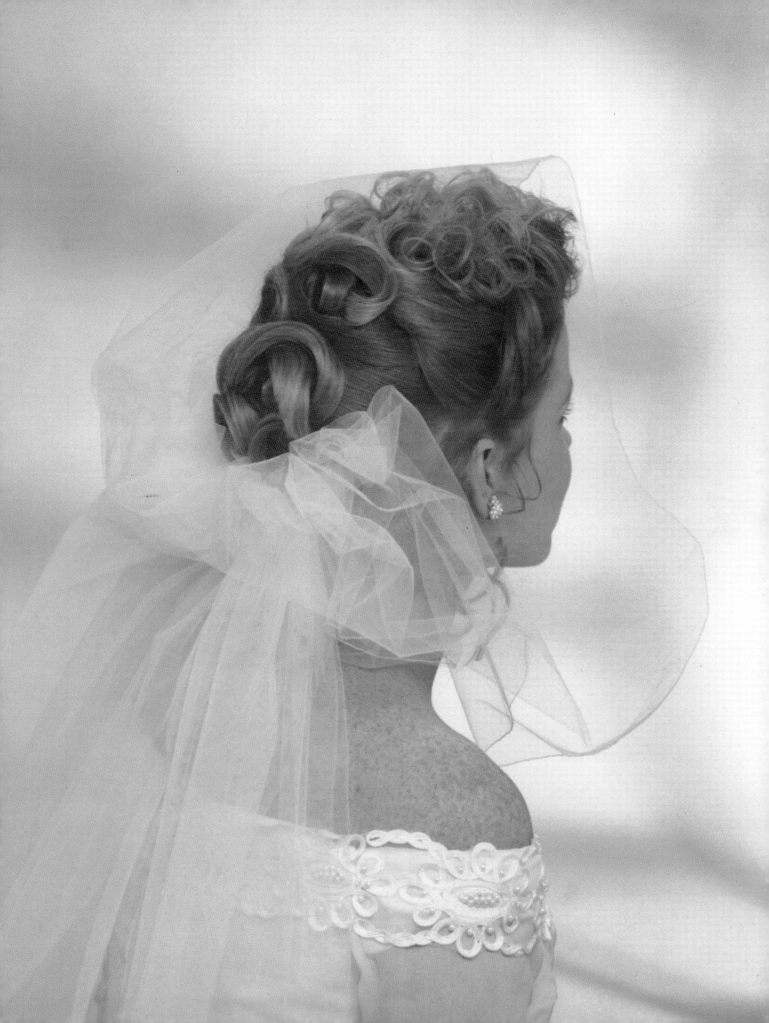

TIARA

Curls contrast with smooth lengths for this beautiful style.

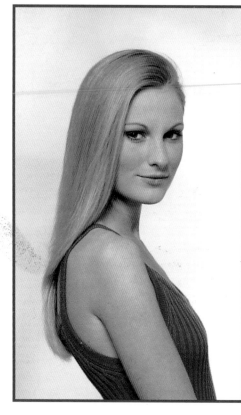

Before

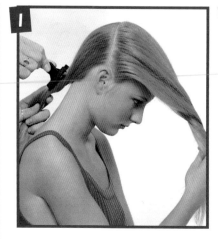

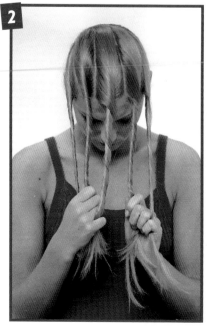

1. Section off top and twist back hair, securing with a clip.

2. Divide front hair into five equal sections and twist each one.

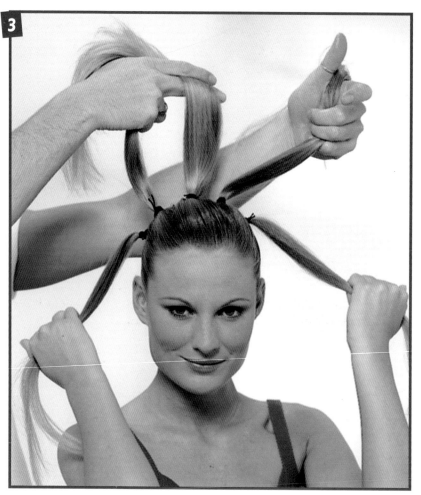

3. Secure each section in a ponytail at crown.

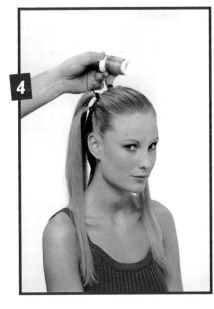

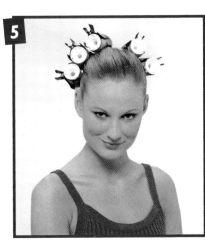

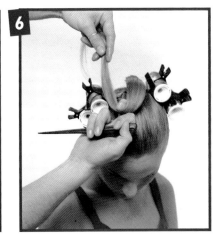

4. Mist each ponytail with a light protective spray and set each one on a heated roller.

5. Leave rollers in place until they are quite cool.

6. Remove one roller at a time. Mist with hairspray to give body and create a silky finish. Twist hair round finger.

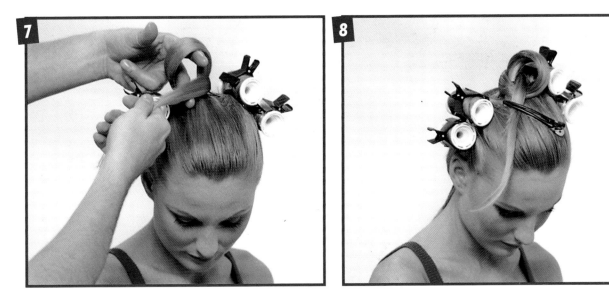

7. Wrap hair over and pull the end through centre to form a loose knot that stands proud like a barrel curl.

8. Hold tail in place with a section clip.

9. Remove remaining heated rollers and knot hair in same way.

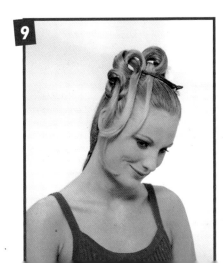

47

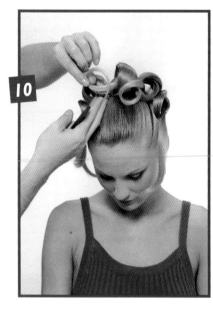

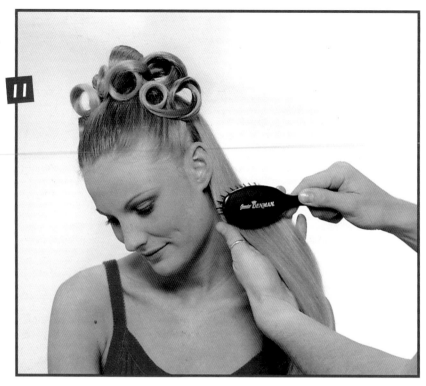

10. Take each tail and form into a barrel curl and pin.

11. Smooth back hair.

12. Add fresh flowers.

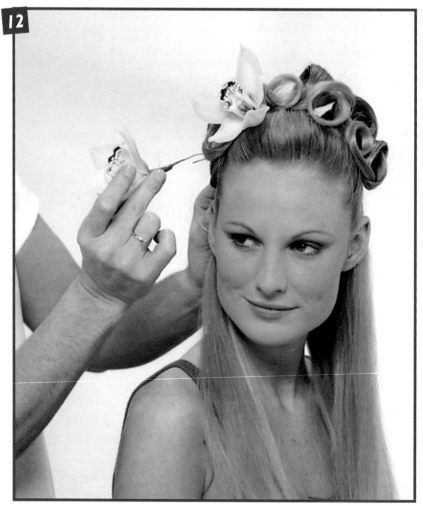

Tip

Ask your florist to wire and bind the ends of each flower so they are easy to fix into hair and don't scratch the scalp.

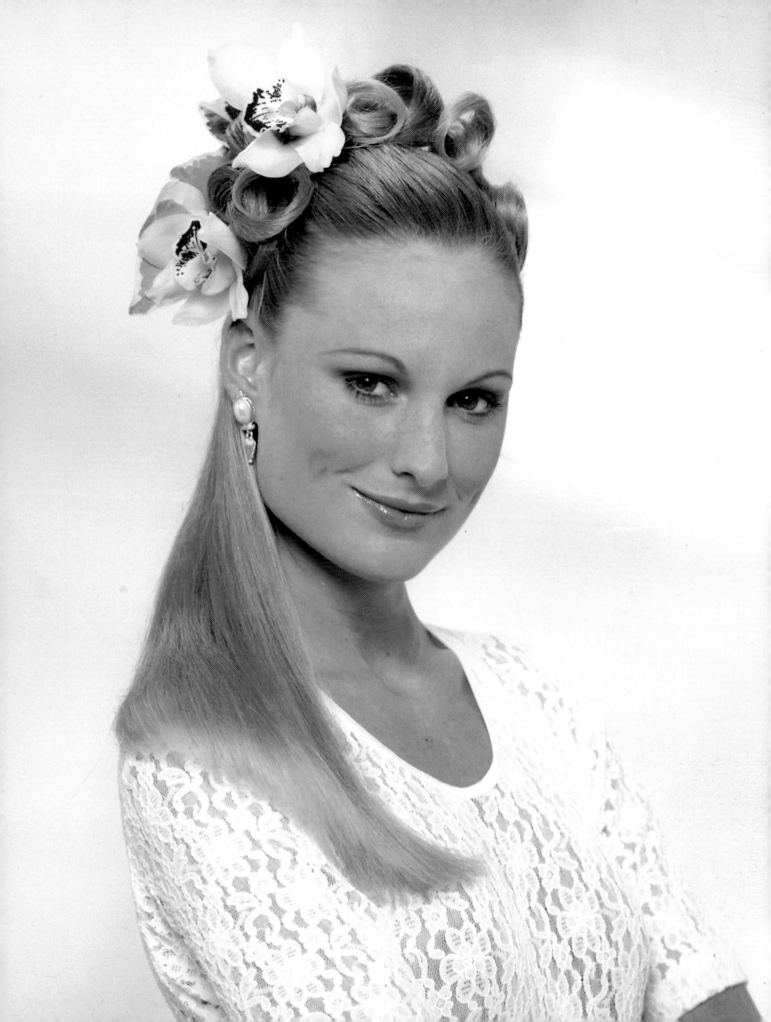

BARREL CURL

Soft curls are intertwined with flowers.

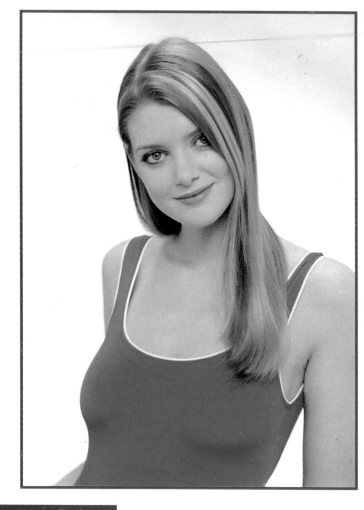

Before

> **❝** Itchy scalps are sensitive so use soothing shampoos and conditioners and soft brushes that gently groom the hair without stressing or irritating the scalp.**❞**

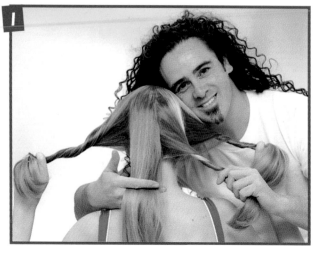

1. Divide hair into four sections.

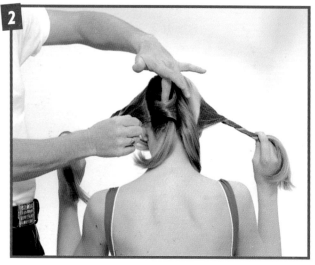

2. Take one section, twist around finger and pin into a barrel-type curl, pin and allow end to fall down onto neck.

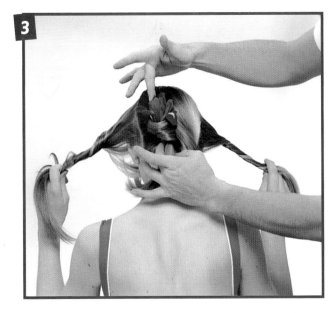

3. Insert flower into centre of barrel curl and pin in place.

4. Repeat with next section of hair.

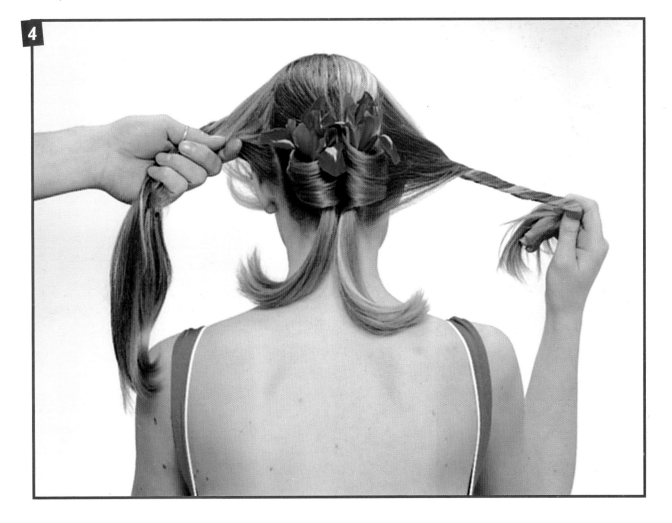

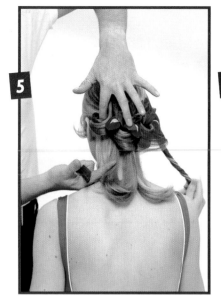

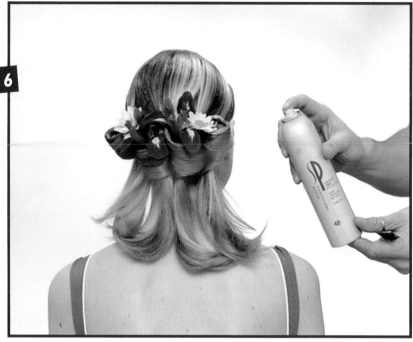

5. Repeat with one side section of hair.

6. Repeat with other side section of hair and mist finished curls with hairspray.

7. Take each of the four ends, curl around finger and pin before adding hair accessories.

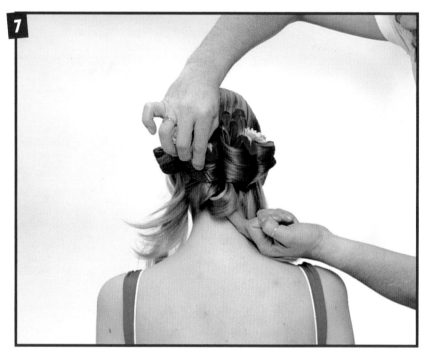

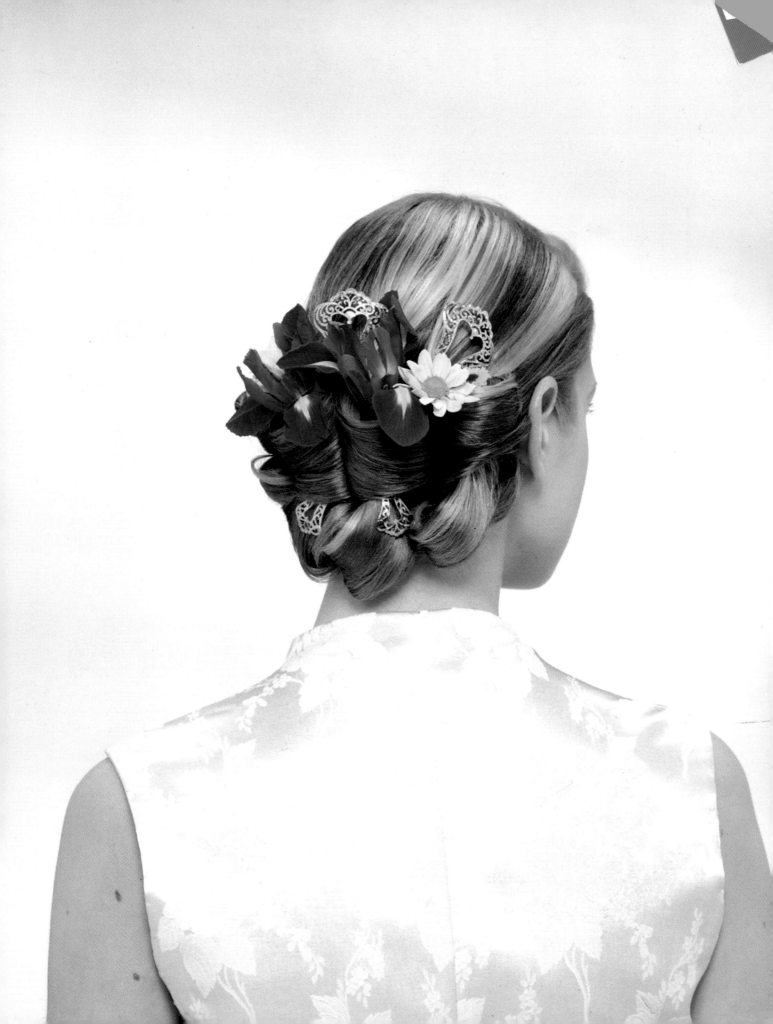

ELIZABETHAN BRAID

Hair drapes into a tiny central braid set off with flowers.

Before

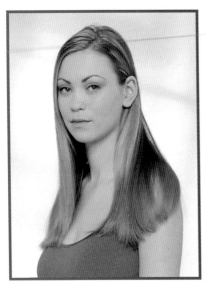

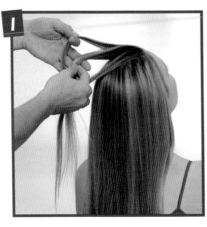

1. Divide off a small triangular section of hair from crown and split into three equal sections.

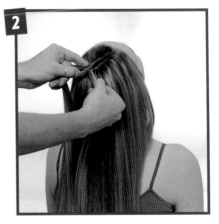

2. Begin braiding by placing left section over right, right section over left.

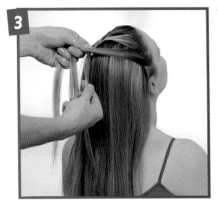

3. Pick up a narrow section of hair from each side at front hairline and work into braid. Braid seven times, before taking another section from each side.

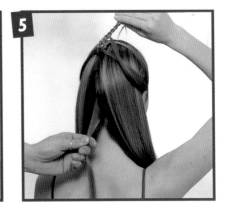

4. Repeat this process – you should have reached approximately half way down the back of the head.

6. Link top braid to this section, continuing the braiding to secure the two pieces of hair together. Comb hair over ends and mist with hairspray. Add flowers.

5. Part back hair and take a small section from nape area at centre back.

Tip
Make sure you hold hair out from head when forming braid to give the style a loose and soft feel.

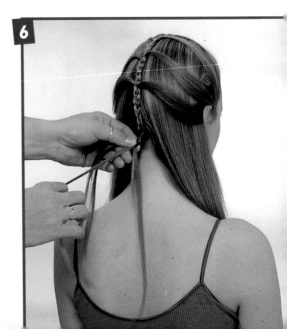

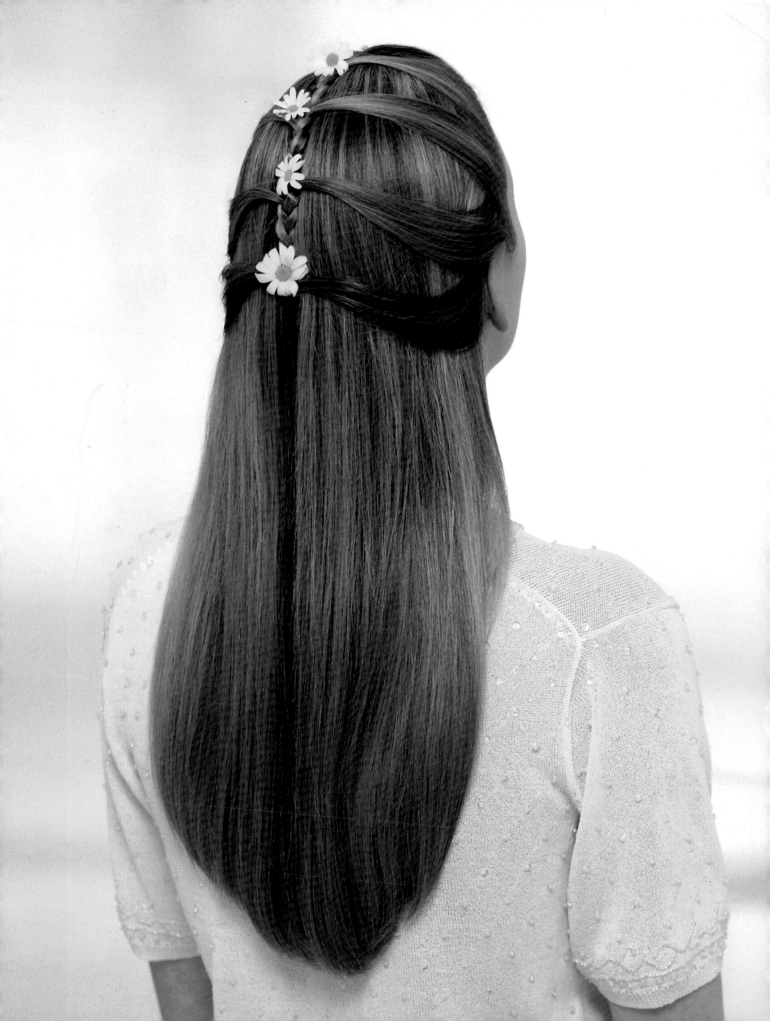

It looks complicated but hair is easily twisted to create this look.

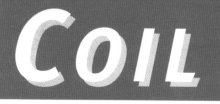

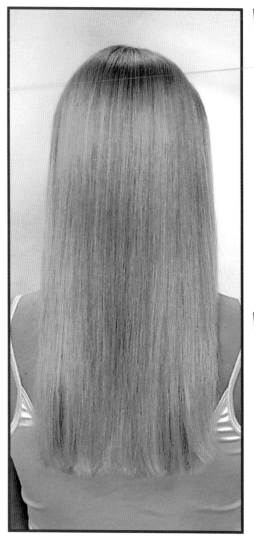

Before

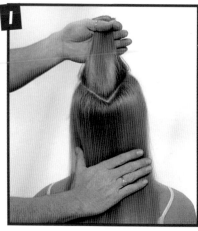

1. Divide off crown hair into a large V-shaped section from left temple down to right temple.

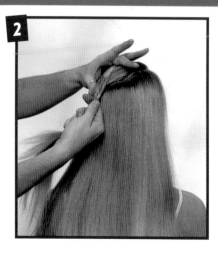

2. Starting from left-hand side, twist hair in a clockwise direction.

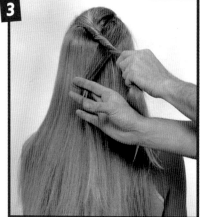

3. Pass twist to right-hand side and prepare to join with a narrow section taken from temple to centre back.

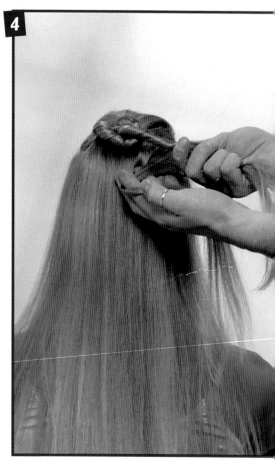

Tip

When twisting hair from side to side it is important that you physically move your whole body weight from one side to the other. Stand to the right shoulder first then the left shoulder and repeat. Keep hair flat to head, do not hold out at an angle or tension will be lost.

4. Continue to twist — you will find that hair begins to coil back on itself.

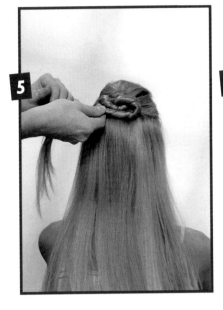

5. Join pieces together and twist back to other side using a clockwise movement.

6. Continue in same manner, going back and forth, adding new hair into the coil at each side and remembering to continue twisting each time you pick up a new section of hair. The right side should go under and left side should go over.

&& Shiatsu head massage is the ultimate in relaxation. Great for revitalising lifeless, stressed-out hair, it is particularly beneficial when treating scalp disorders.&&

7. Repeat until you reach nape of neck. Pin end of final coil in place and insert pearl pins down each side.

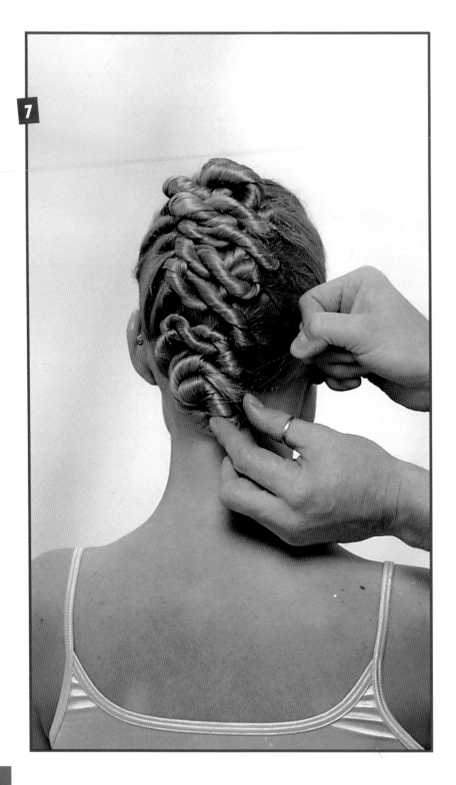

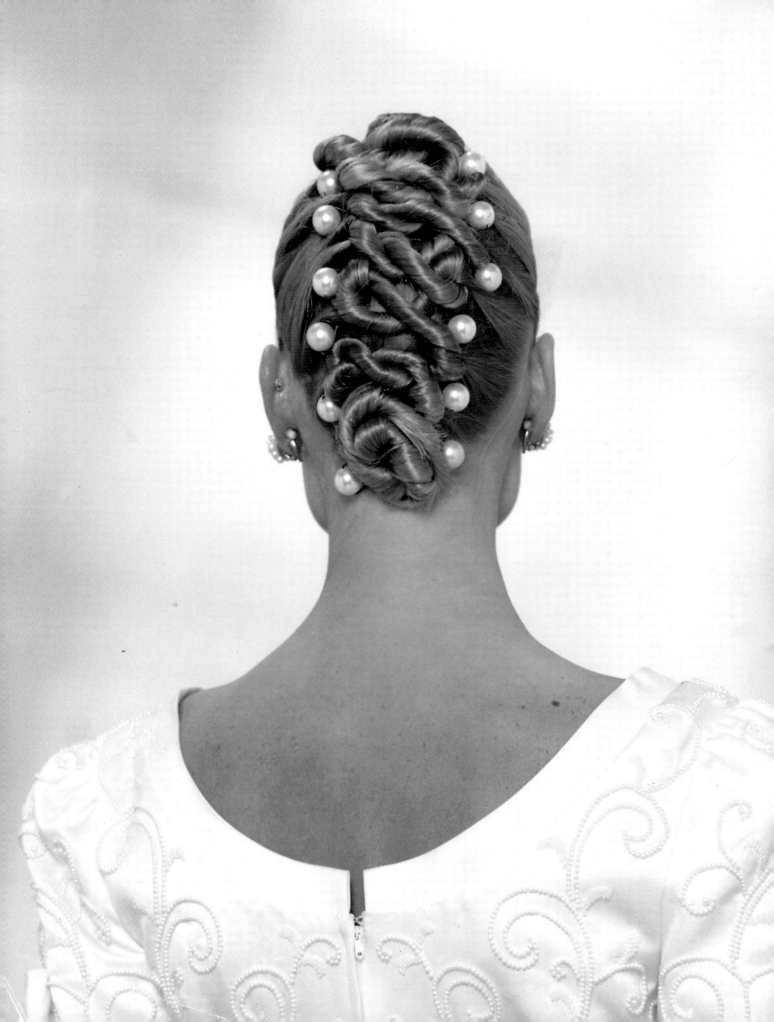

Elegant, Edwardian-inspired style where hair forms into a luxurious loop.

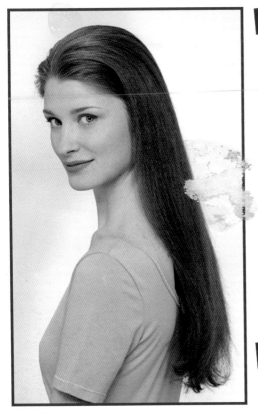

Before

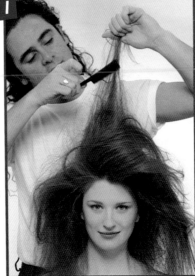

1. Backcomb hair all over.

> 66 Ultra-violet sterilisation is used in salons to disinfect brushes and combs. At home, wash your styling equipment in warm, soapy water and leave to dry naturally. 99

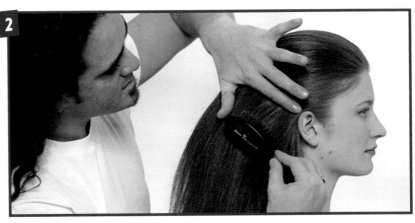

2. Smooth hair over, flat to head, using a bristle brush.

3. Place a row of criss-crossed grips around the back of head.

4. Divide hair into three sections.

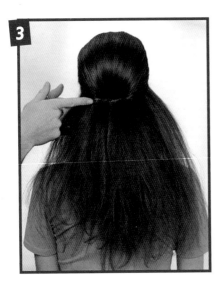

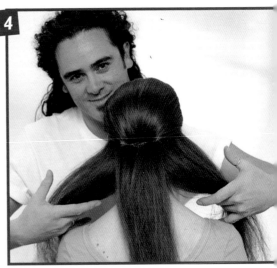

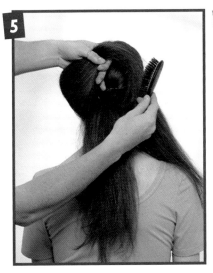

5. Take one side section of hair, smooth with a bristle brush and roll hair over hand.

6. Fold ends downwards so a large loop is formed.

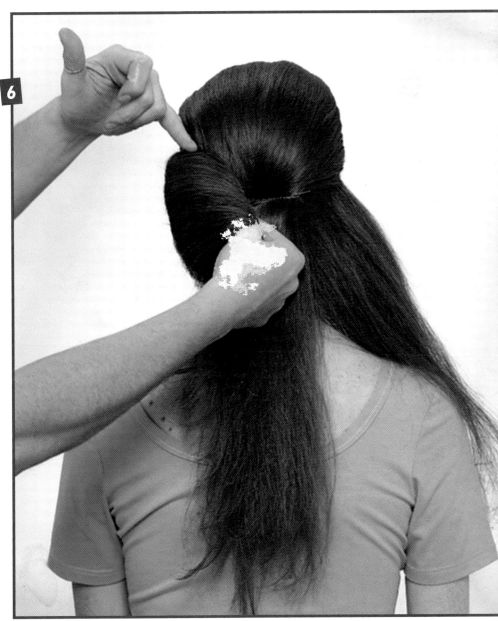

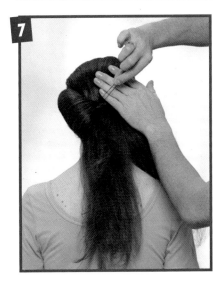

7. Pin in position.

8. Repeat for other side making sure you leave a 2.5 cm gap in centre.

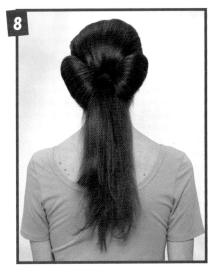

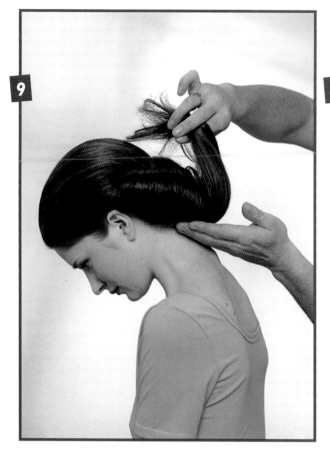

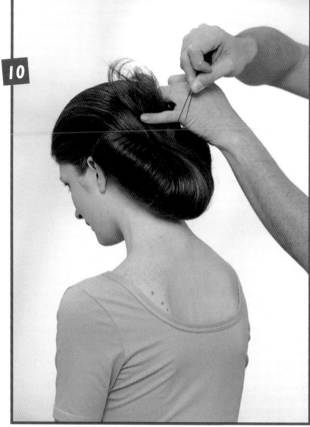

9. Take centre back section of hair and fold upwards into a roll.

10. Pin at centre back.

11. Swirl ends into a flat pincurl, secure with a hairgrip and add fresh flowers.

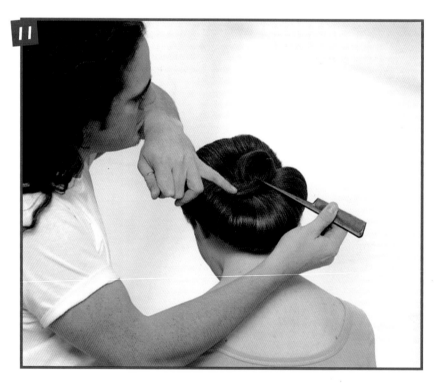

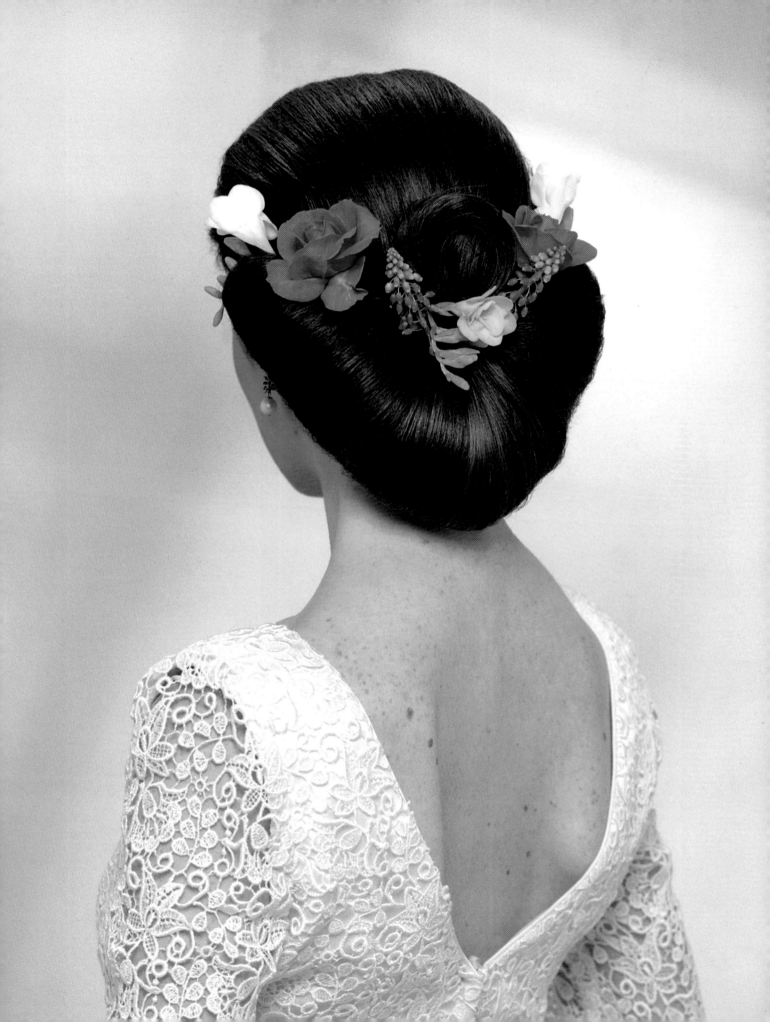

LOW ROLL

A low ponytail quickly transforms into this classic style.

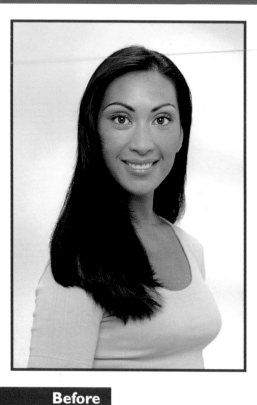

1. Keeping fringe free, use a bristle brush to smooth remaining hair into low ponytail.

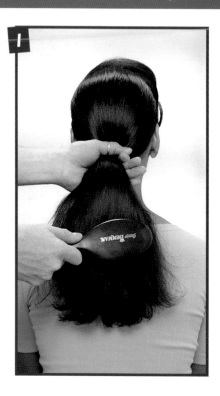

❝ Thick hair can be tamed if you use an air-cushion bristle brush with nylon quills which penetrates through the hair helping to spread the natural oils along the hair shaft evenly to give sheen, lustre and control. ❞

2. Backcomb ponytail.

3. Using a bristle brush, smooth over top layer of back-combed ponytail and mist with hairspray.

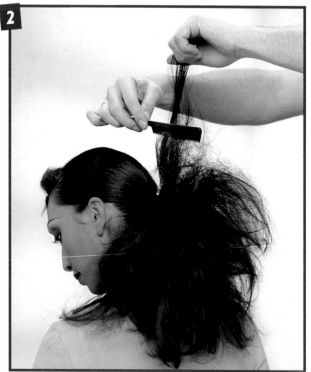

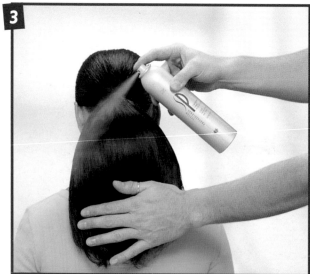

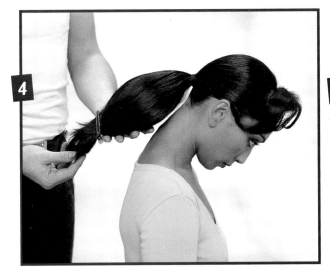

4. Secure ends of ponytail with a section clip.

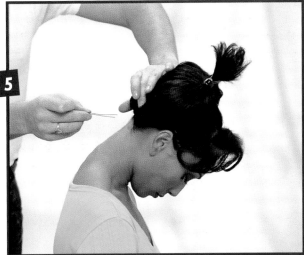

5. Flip ponytail up onto crown and place overlapping grips around base in a horseshoe fashion. These should be approximately 1 cm from ponytail. This forms base for bun and gives stability.

6. Flip ponytail back over.

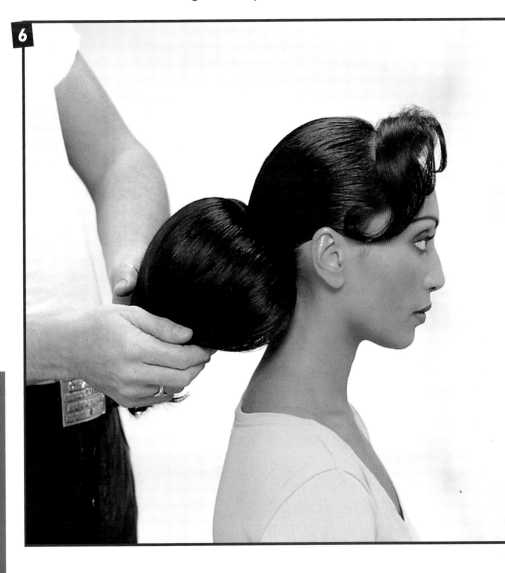

Tip

When removing back-combing, use a wide-toothed comb and work from ends upwards to roots then smooth through using a bristle brush.

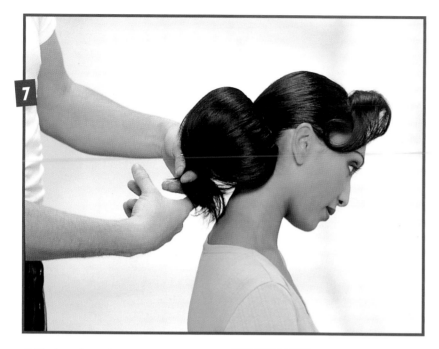

7. Tuck ends under.

8. Pin in place. Backcomb and smooth fringe.

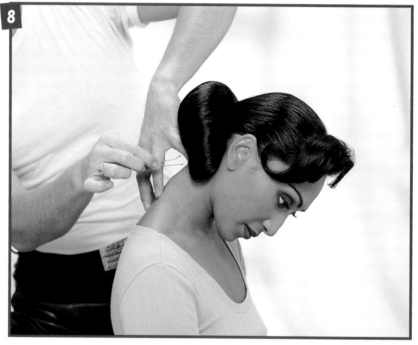

Newly washed hair is easier to handle and put up if you smooth a little styling lotion through the lengths first.

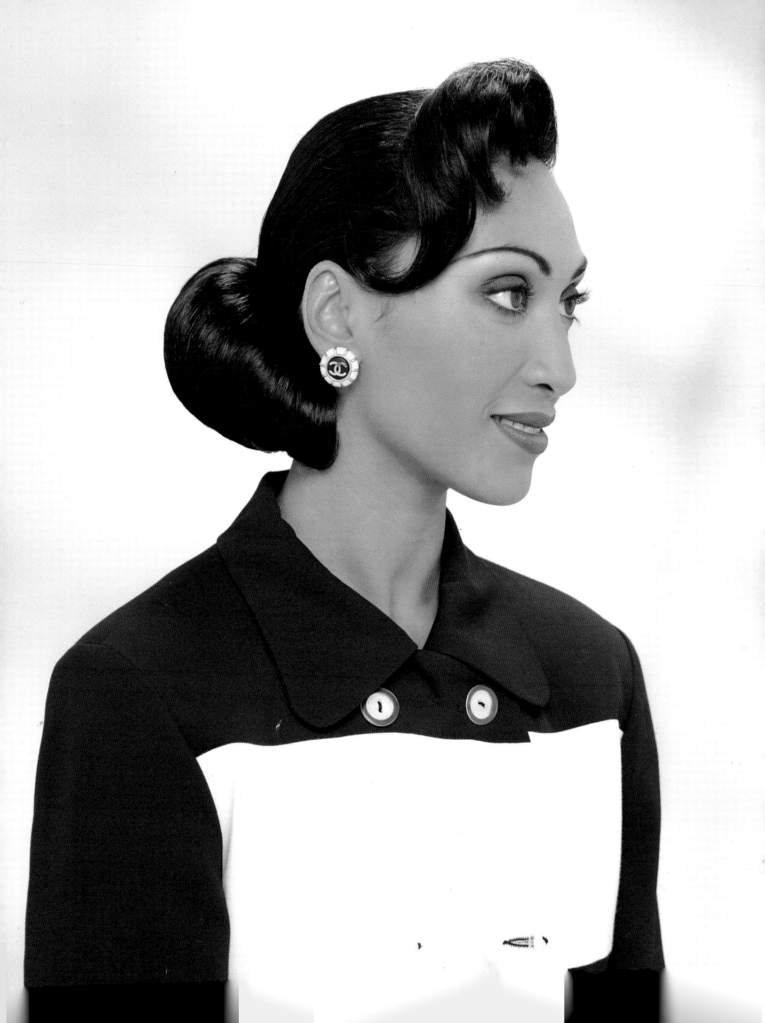

SOFT ROLL

Natural curls are controlled without losing their femininity.

Before

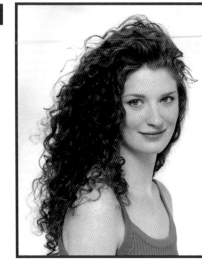

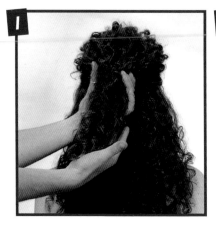

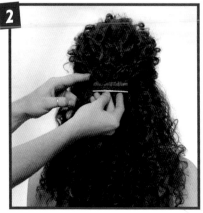

1. Use fingers to section off top and side hair.

2. Secure using a diamanté comb or similar.

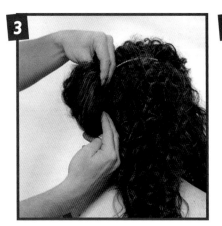

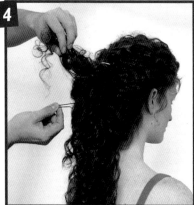

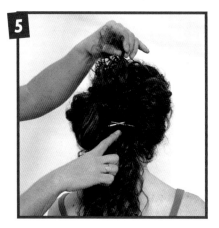

3. Separate hair into three sections. Take one side section and roll towards centre back. Secure with a hairgrip. Repeat for other side.

4. Lift up top hair and insert hairgrips.

5. Crossed hairgrips at centre back of head form the base for lower hair when it is rolled up.

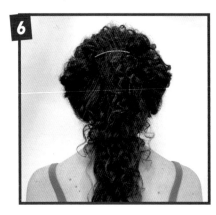

6. Let top hair fall back down to cover grips.

7. Clip top hair out of the way, then roll lower hair up and over the crossed hairgrips and secure with pins. Lower the top hair back over the roll to create a soft curl effect before pinning head-dress in place.

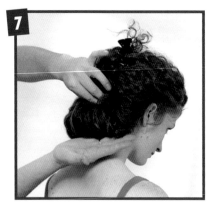

68

Tip
Don't brush natural curls. Rake through with fingers or use a wide-toothed comb.

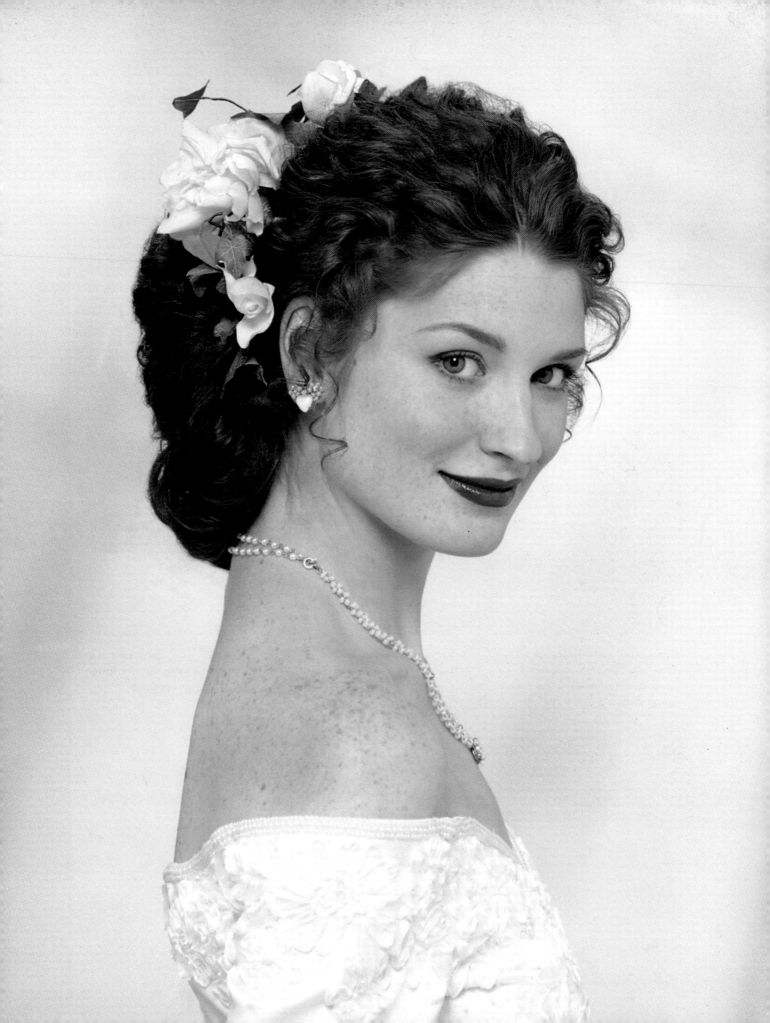

TOP ROLL
A halo of hair is set off with a tiara.

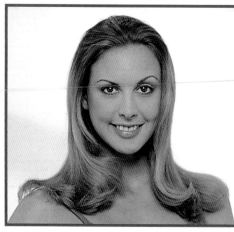

Before

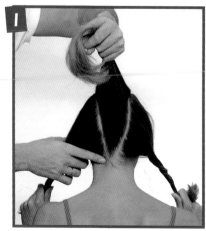

1. Part hair in a V shape from front hairline to centre nape.

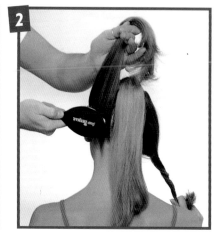

2. Secure top hair at crown in a band and brush one side section upwards to just below first ponytail. Leave a small section of hair free at each side for curling later.

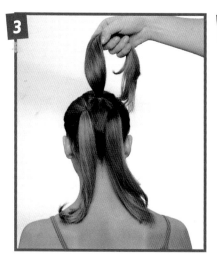

3. Secure in a band and repeat for other side. The two side ponytails are lower than the top one.

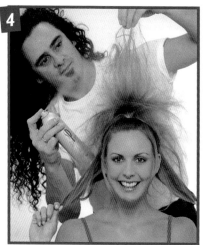

4. Backcomb middle ponytail and mist with hairspray.

Tip
This shape can be made larger or smaller depending on how tightly each ponytail is folded.

5. Smooth with a bristle brush, secure ends with section clip.

6. Flip backcombed ponytail over to front and and pin with a row of grips, 2.5 cm from band.

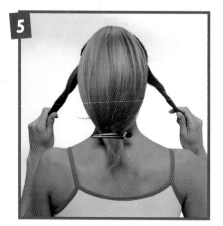

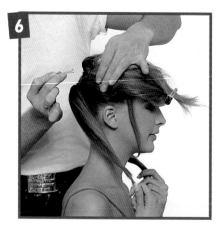

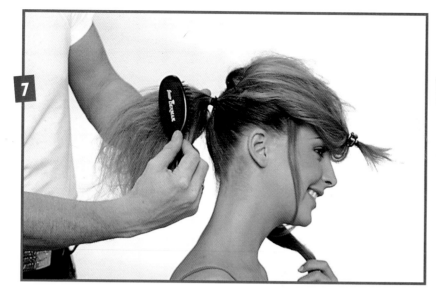

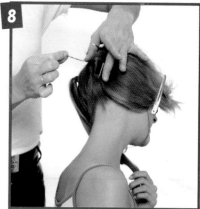

7. Backcomb one side ponytail, mist with hairspray and smooth over.

8. Secure end in section clip, flip to front and insert grips as before. Repeat for other side.

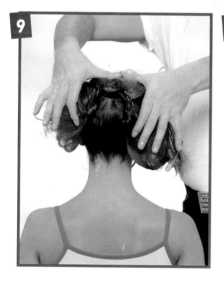

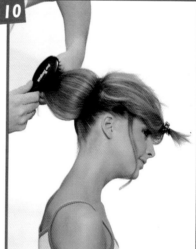

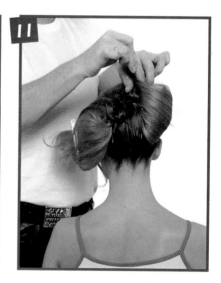

9. Shows completed side sections clipped and held forward.

10. Smooth one side section around hand.

11. Roll side section round fingers smoothing into palm of hand. Twist upwards into a cone shape. Spray and secure with vertically placed hairpins. Coil ends into top of cone.

12. Twist ends in and pin. Repeat for other side, making sure cones are symmetrical. If necessary, use ends of a tailcomb to sleek in any wisps of hair.

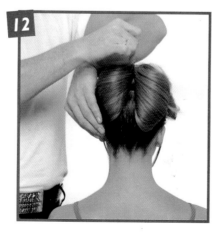

13. Take front section and re-smooth.

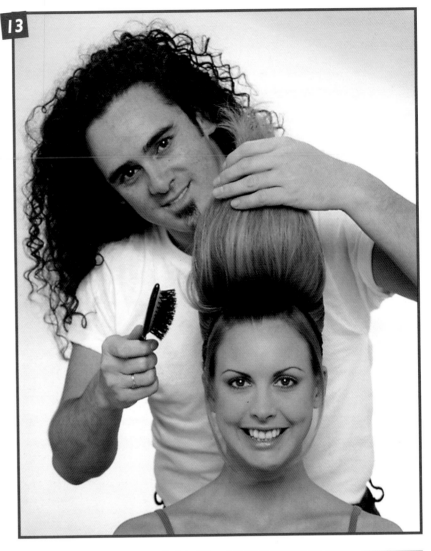

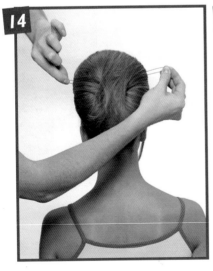

14. Place hair centrally, blending over back coils as you sweep back and pin. Make sure you keep an eye on the shape and balance.

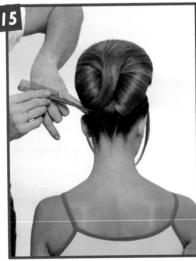

15. Smooth ends into a loose curl which covers the hairpins at back. Neaten ends using a tailcomb.

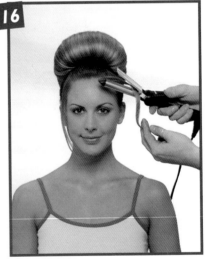

16. Tong side hair. Re-smooth top hair if necessary and mist with hair-spray before adding a pearl and diamanté tiara.

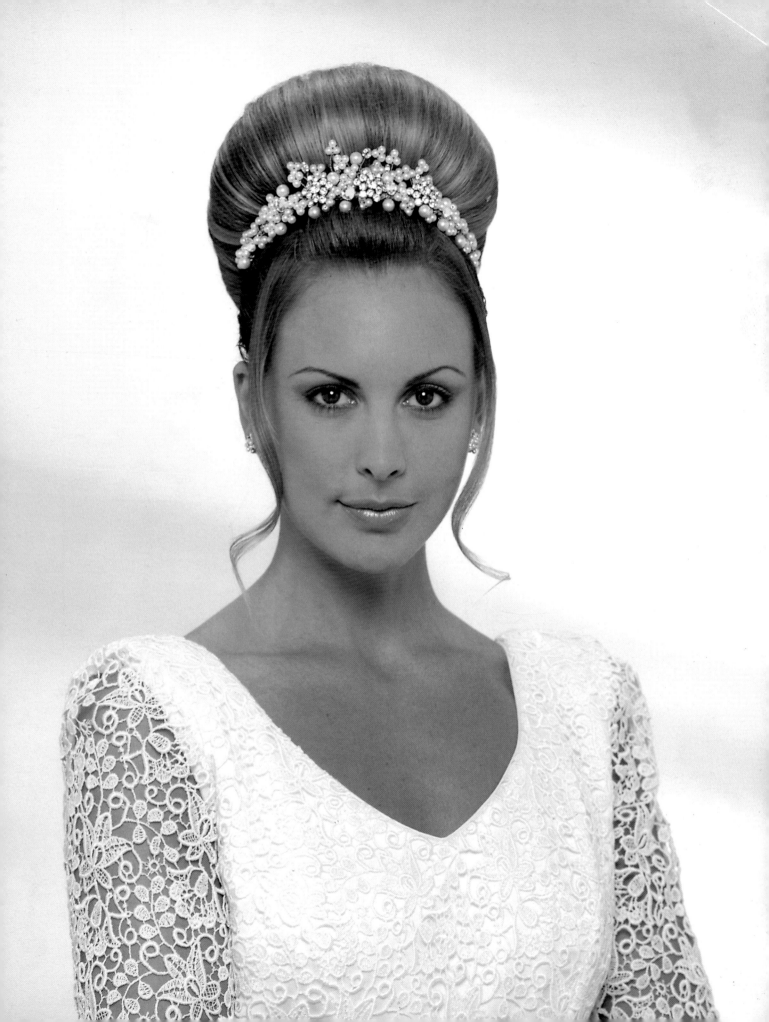

Hair is swirled and curled to create this demure look.

Before

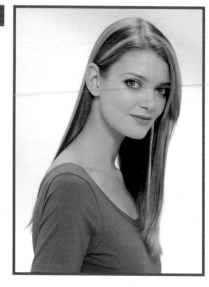

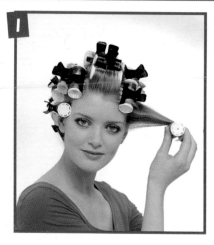

1. Mist hair with styling lotion and set on heated rollers.

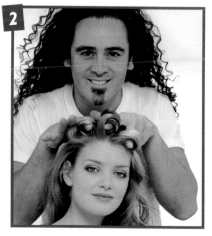

2. Remove rollers and set front hair in three barrel curls, pin in place.

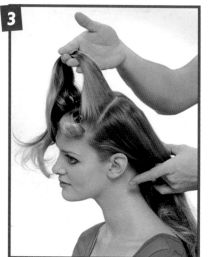

3. Divide off a triangular section on crown and place into a section clip.

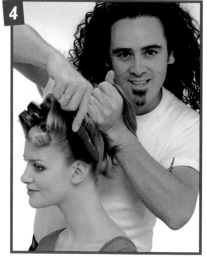

4. Brush hair smoothly back.

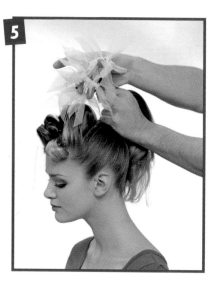

5. Use a band that has been tied with strips of ribbon.

6. Pull hair through band.

Tip

This style is perfect for those who prefer not to have any backcombing in their hair. Misting each section with hairspray as you work makes the hair more malleable and holds style for longer.

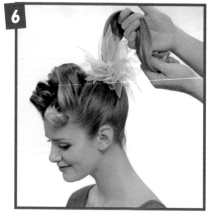

7. Take reserved triangular section of hair and smooth back.

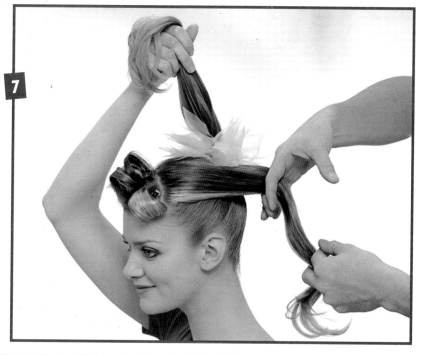

8. Use a tailcomb to curve hair into an S shape and grip in place.

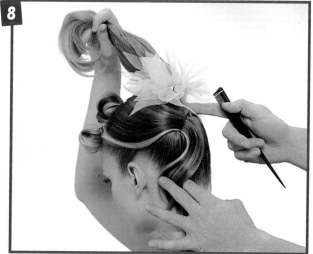

9. Smooth ponytail into loop and pin as shown

10. Twist tail end into a flat pincurl and secure.

11. Shows ponytail pinned in position.

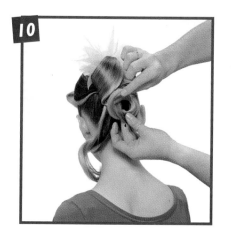

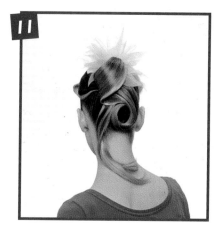

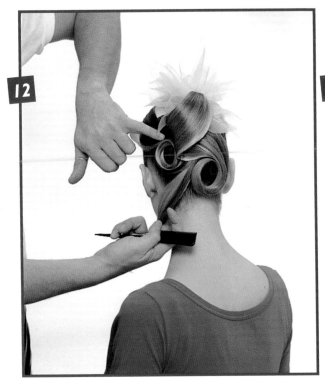

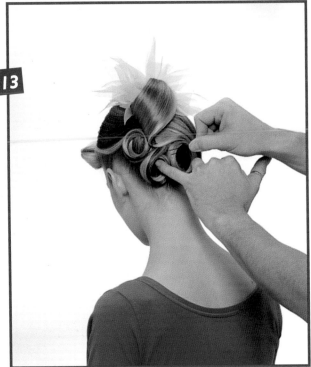

12. Take remaining piece of hair, divide into two and form top section into a flat pincurl and secure.

13. Form lower section into a flat pincurl and secure.

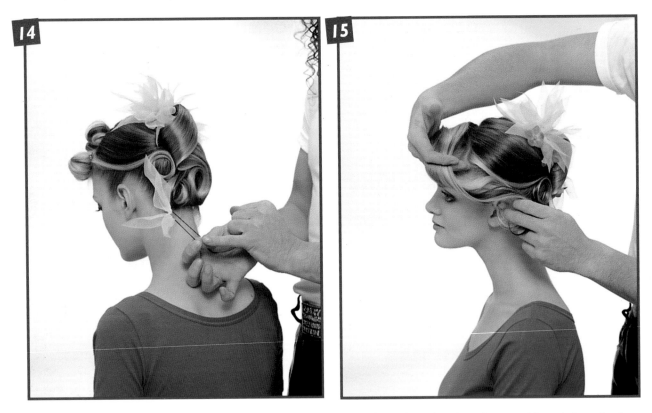

14. Tie a piece of ribbon onto a large hairpin and insert at centre back.

15. Release barrel curls at front and loop hair to back, forming end into another flat pin curl. Secure and add fresh flowers.

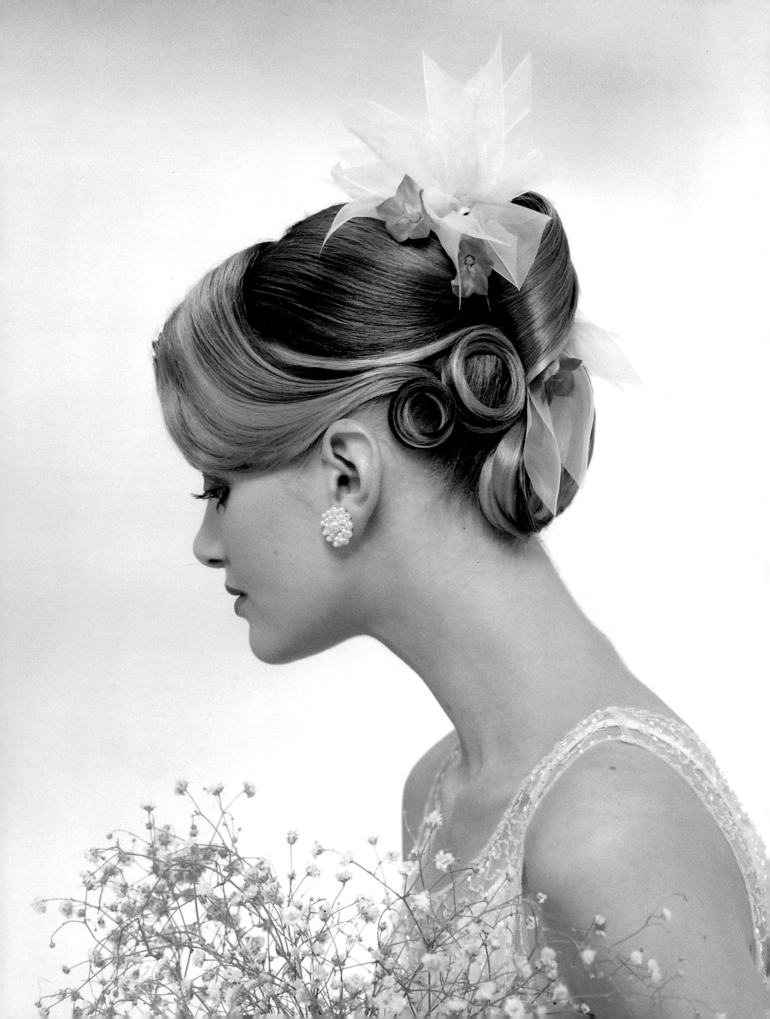

Bow

Hair is sculpted into shape so it resembles a ribbon.

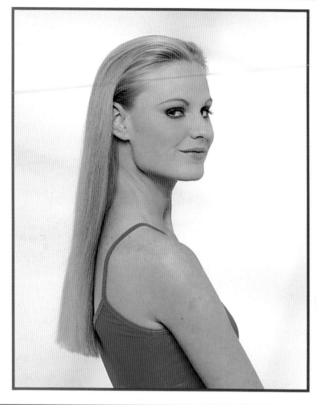

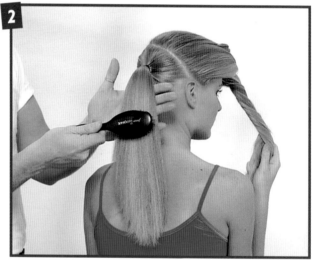

1. Divide hair into two sections of roughly the same bulk.

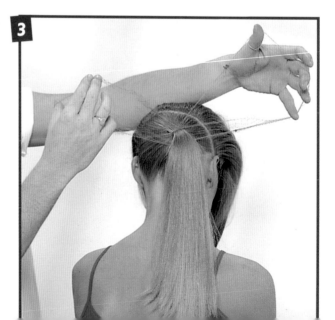

2. Brush back hair into a ponytail which should be positioned just off the centre of the back of the head.

Tip

When dividing hair into two sections for this style you should literally 'feel the weight' in your hands so you ensure an equal balance for finished bow.

3. Fix two hairnets to base of ponytail.

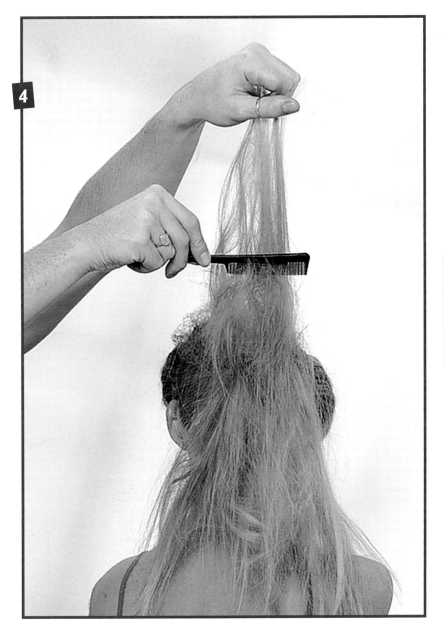

4

4. Backcomb ponytail.

5. Use a bristle brush to smooth ponytail.

6. Mist ponytail with hairspray.

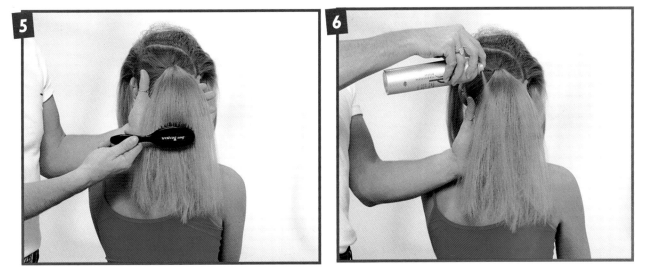

5

6

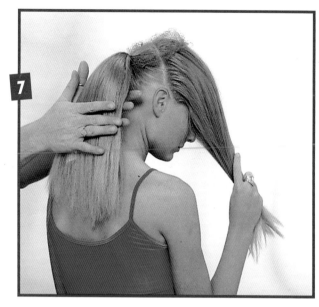

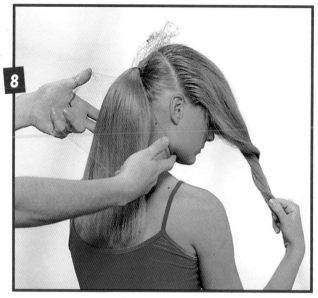

7. Press hair between palms to make it smooth and flat like a ribbon.

8. Lower net over smoothed ponytail.

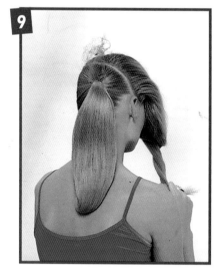

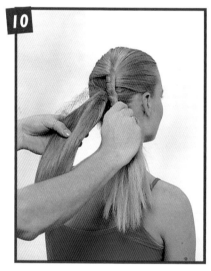

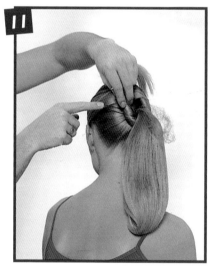

9. Shows ponytail in net.

10. Brush top hair back and over to one side. Twist in a clockwise direction and take twist under first ponytail.

12. Backcomb tail end of this section.

11. Loop upwards and pin.

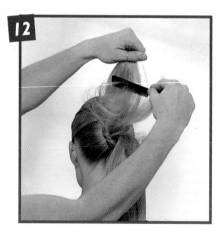

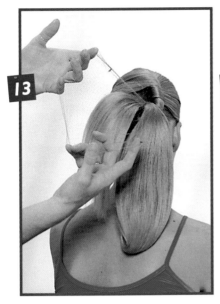

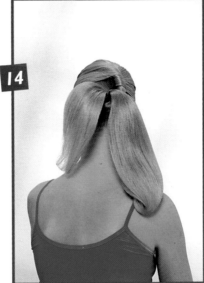

13. Smooth end of hair with a bristle brush and apply hairspray as before. Then twist net round and take it over this section of hair.

14. Shows netted ponytails.

15. Roll netted ponytail round fingers at a 45° angle – if you do not get the angle right the shape will not mirror a perfect bow.

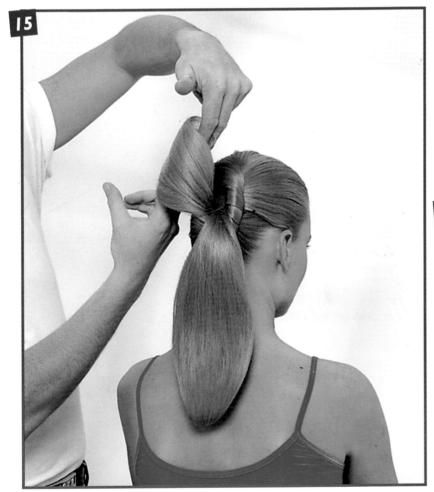

16. Pin roll in place.

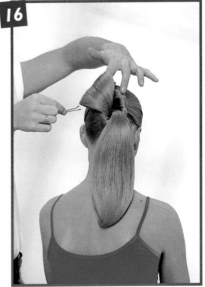

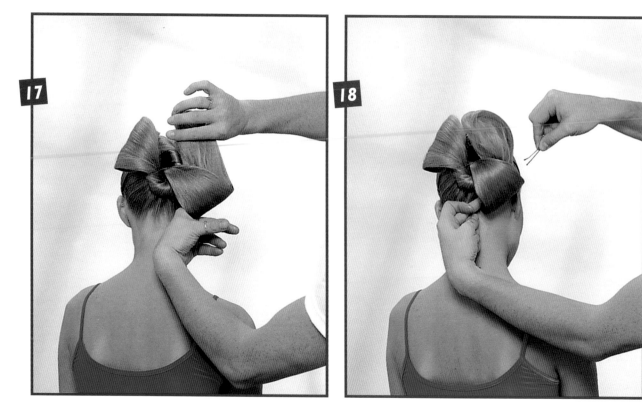

17. Roll other netted ponytail round fingers in same manner.

18. Pin in place through centre of roll.

19. Take tail end over and tuck in.

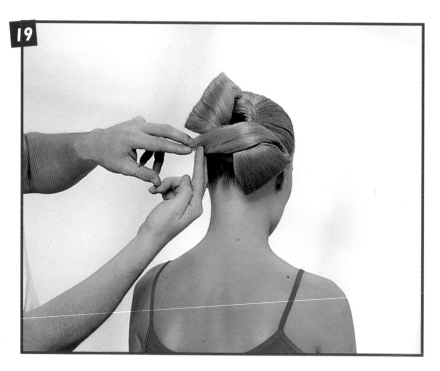

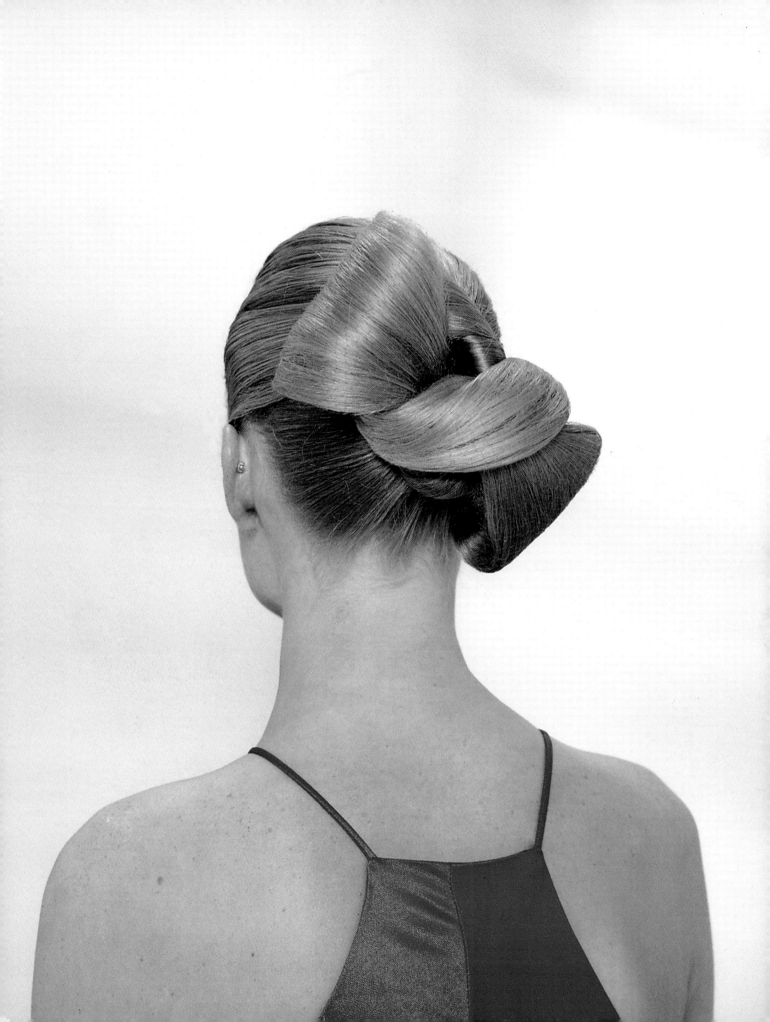

TIFFANY

A ponytail is swirled with hair to give this classic style.

Before

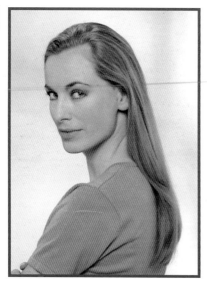

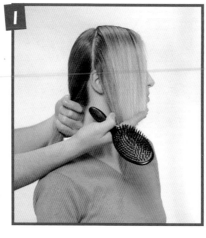

1. Part hair from ear to ear and divide off front section.

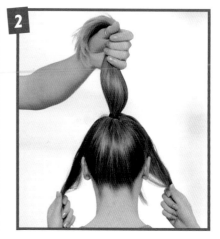

2. Brush back hair up into a high ponytail.

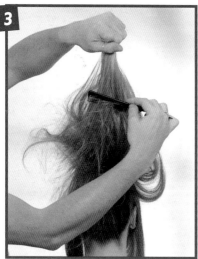

3. Backcomb ponytail.

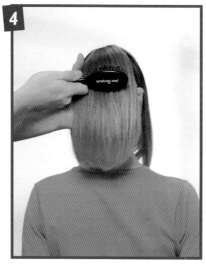

4. Smooth over top layer of ponytail using a bristle brush.

6. Flip ponytail to left side and insert a grip upwards, 2 cm from ponytail.

7. Fold ponytail back over to other side, holding with fingers.

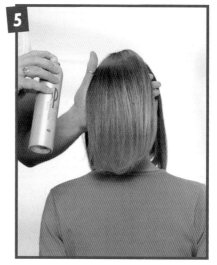

5. Mist with hairspray.

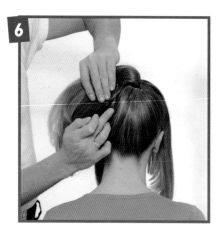

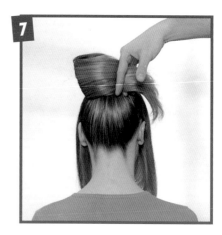

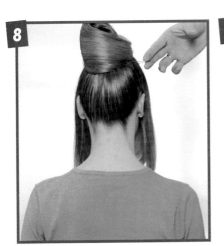

8. Pin to secure.

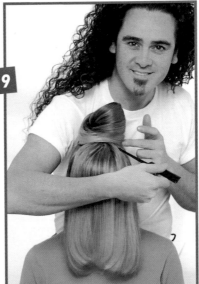

9. Use a tailcomb to tuck in any stray ends.

Tip

When brushing hair around, make sure it wraps following the flow of the previously positioned hair so that it forms a swirl.

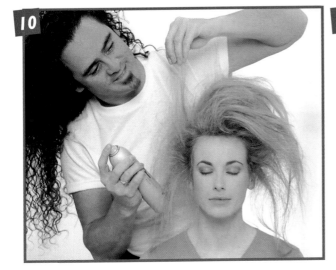
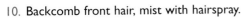

10. Backcomb front hair, mist with hairspray.

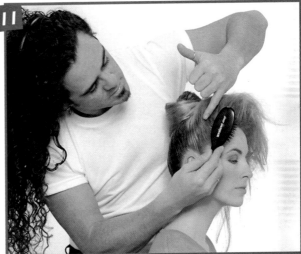

11. Gently smooth to one side using a bristle brush in the same direction as the back fold.

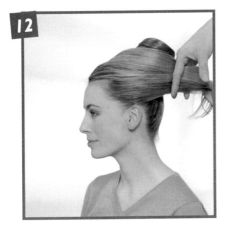

12. Take hair round bun, holding the section flat and wide (3–4 cm) between fingers.

13. Pin in place.

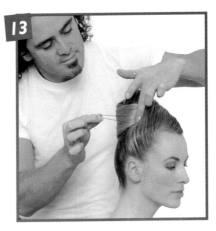

14. Neaten ends with tailcomb before fixing veil and rosebuds in place. If veil is creased, simply blast with a hairdryer whilst shaking out.

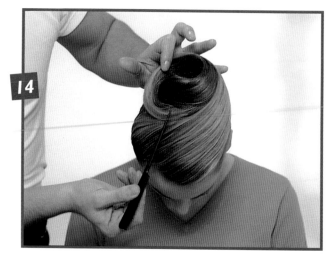

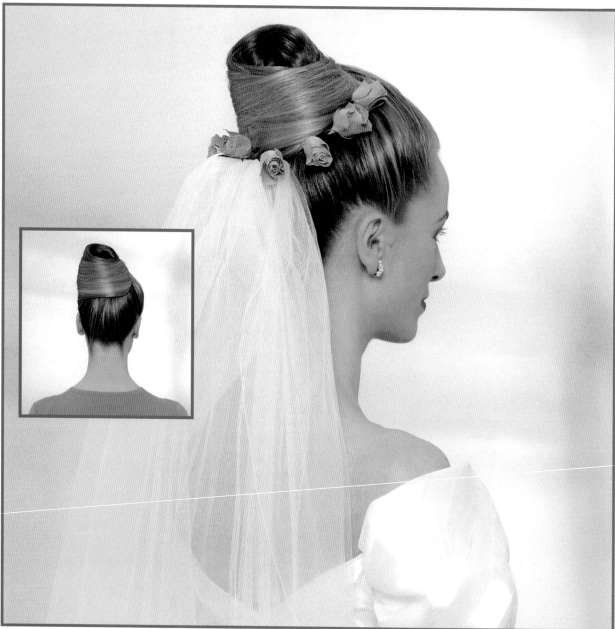

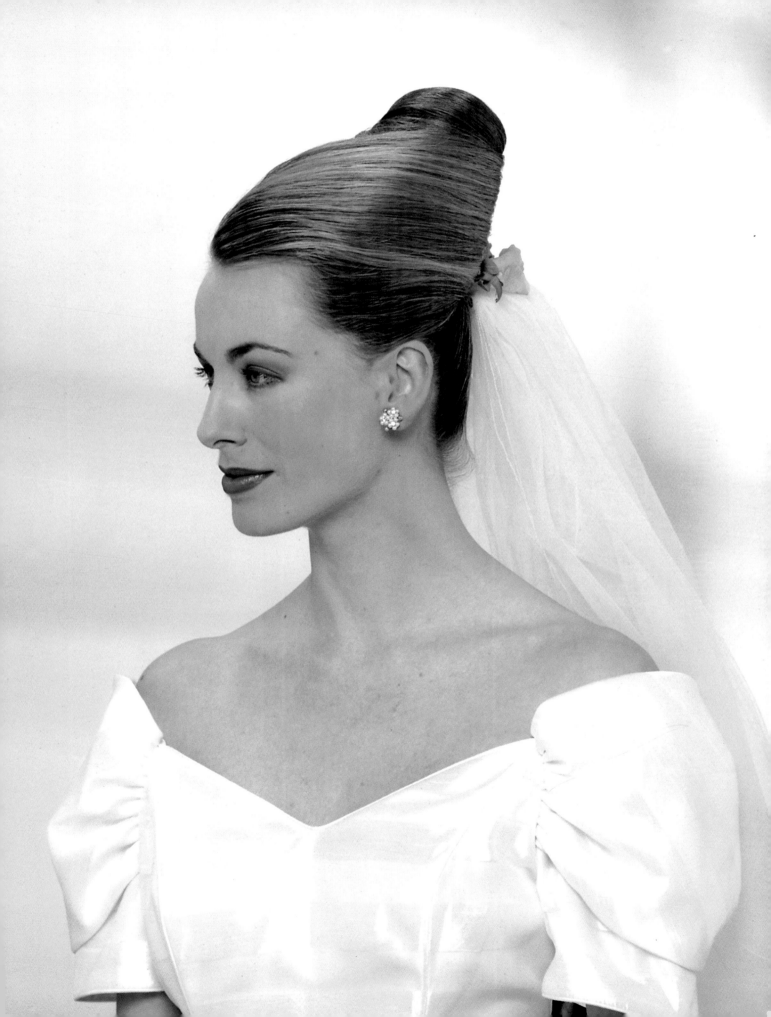

FRENCH PLEAT

This timeless style is easy to achieve if you work methodically.

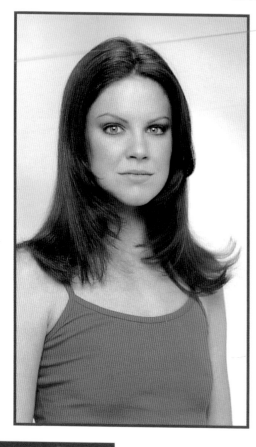

Before

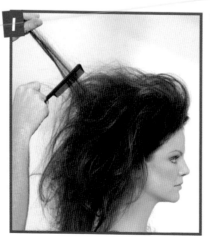

1. Backcomb hair and mist with hairspray.

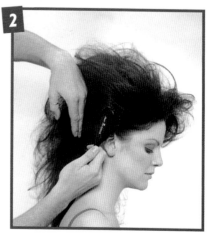

2. Smooth using a bristle brush.

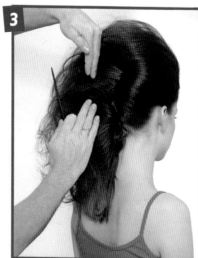

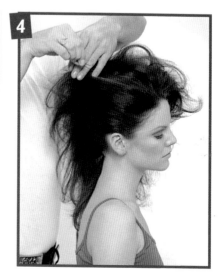

3. Insert a row of grips up centre back of head.

4. Begin smoothing top hair.

5. Divide off lower section of hair from lobe of ear. Position hand vertically as shown to keep flat.

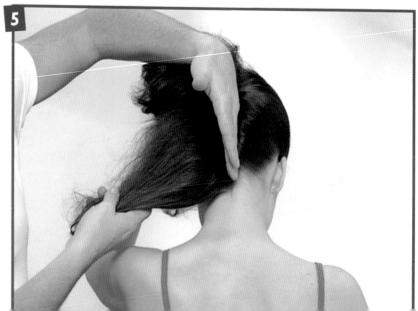

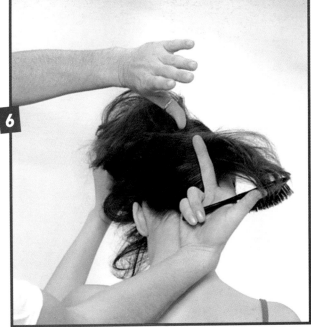

6. Wrap hair over.

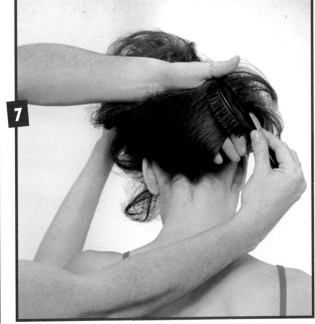

7. Smoothing with bristle brush.

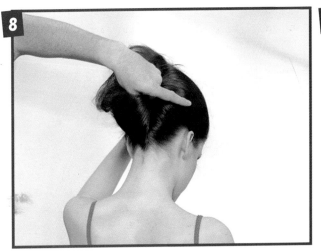

8. Twist hair around thumb using an upward movement so the ends of the twist are placed following the line of grips. Pin grips vertically down seam of roll. *Do not* insert horizontally into roll.

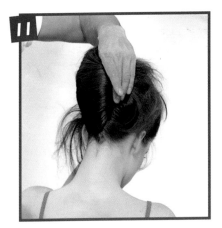

9. Use tailcomb to tuck ends up and into pleat. Do not push down into first section or you will make it too heavy.

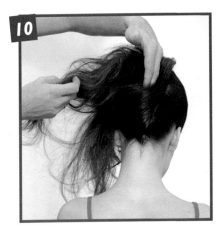

10. Take central section of hair from front temple to crown and brush smooth as before.

11. Mould this section into the previous one, taking ends in as before.

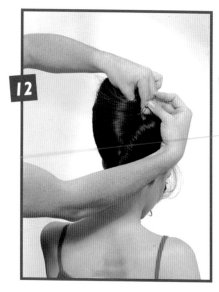

12. Pin downwards as before.

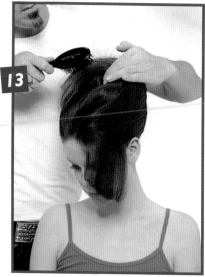

13. To finish top area, brush around and join top ends to those of the two sections and swirl round to finish.

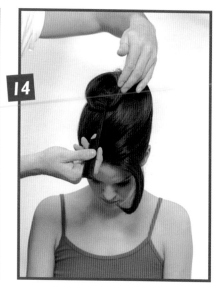

14. Use a tailcomb to flick final ends into a curl and pin.

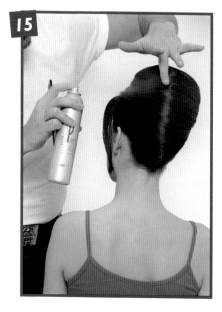

15. Mist with hairspray.

Tip
Hold finished look with a fine mist of shine-enhancing hairspray.

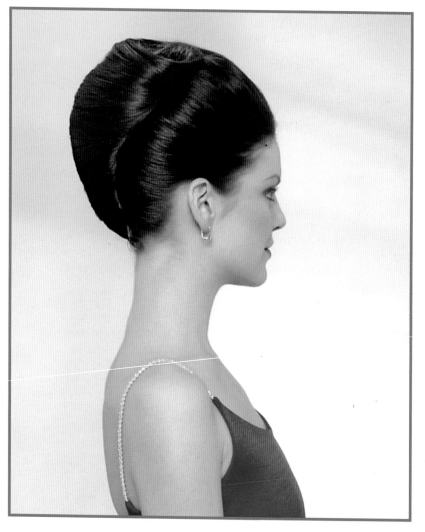

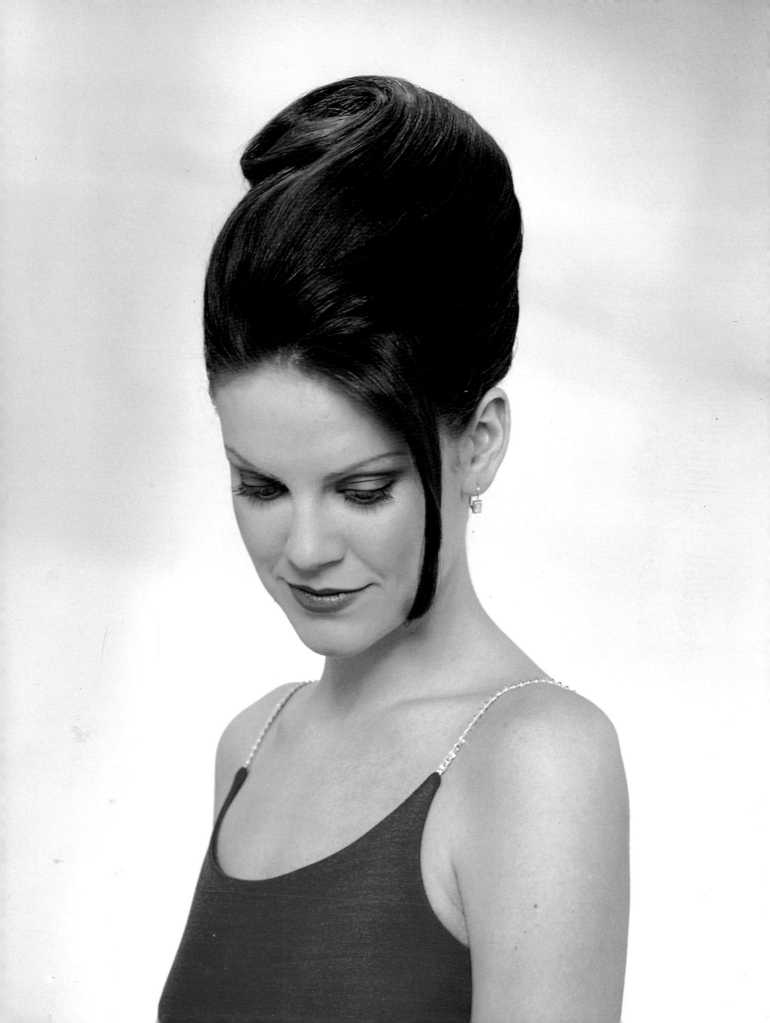

ALTERNATIVE PLEAT

Conical shaping gives a new twist to the traditional pleat.

Before

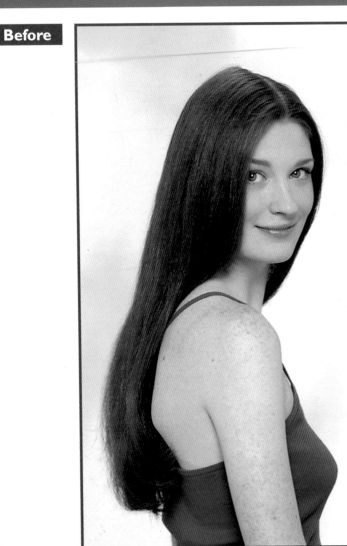

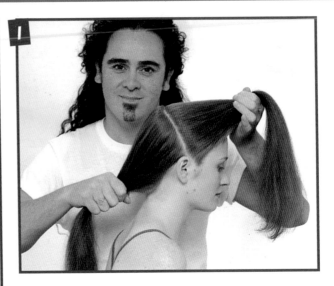

1. Divide hair into front and back sections making parting from ear to ear.

> ❝ Long hair should be trimmed at least every 3 months to keep ends neat and prevent splitting. Intensive weekly deep-conditioning treatments will also help to keep hair healthy and shiny.❞

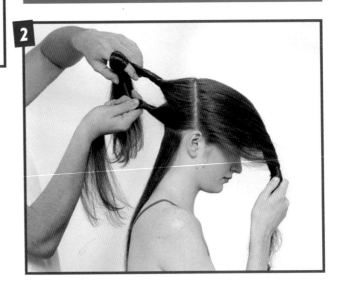

2. Divide back hair into three equal sections.

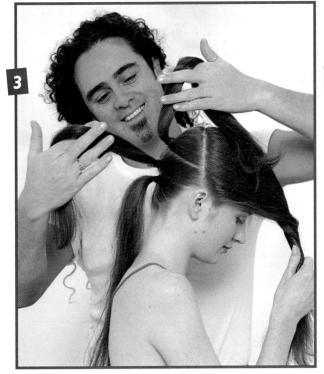

3. Secure ponytails down centre back making sure bottom one is lifted quite high so it is almost taken to top of its section.

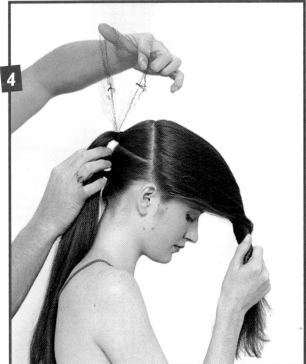

4. Fix net to top ponytail.

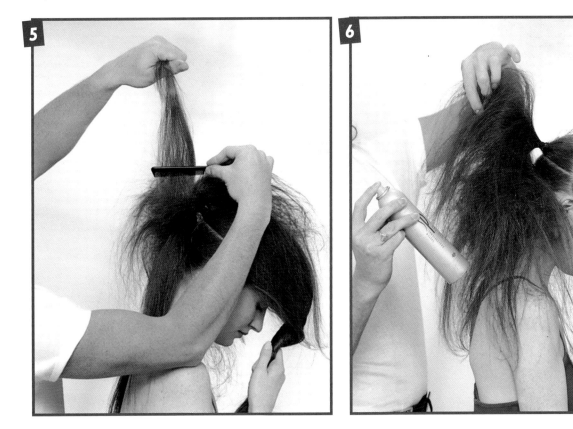

5. Backcomb the three ponytails.

6. Mist hair with hairspray.

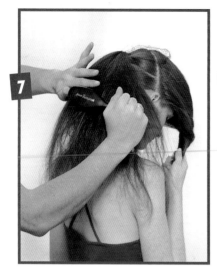

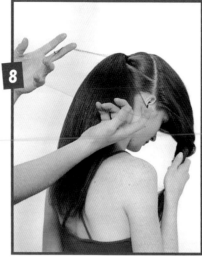

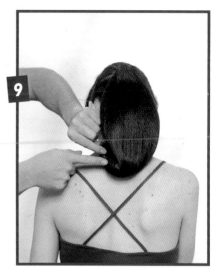

7. Smooth top layer of hair with a bristle brush.

8. Bring net down over all of the hair.

9. Tuck in ends of hair making sure it loops into a large pincurl shape.

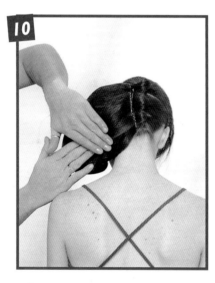

10. Fold hair to one side and secure using a line of crossed hairgrips approximately 1 cm from ponytails.

11. Fold hair back on itself and twist up.

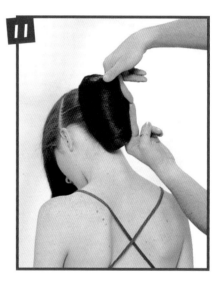

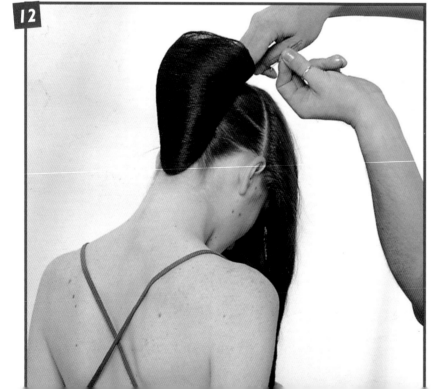

12. Form into a cone using fingers to create shape and grip vertically downwards. The pleat should sit low on the neck so that it gives a curved line that covers the hairline.

Tip

When brushing front hair back it is important to position it around back section following same direction as the roll.

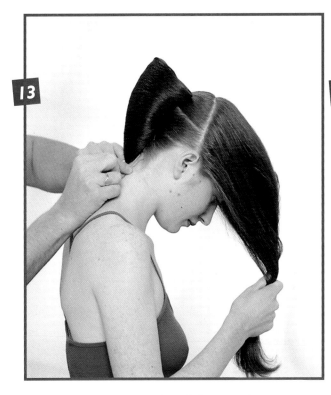

13. Grip vertically upwards and downwards to secure.

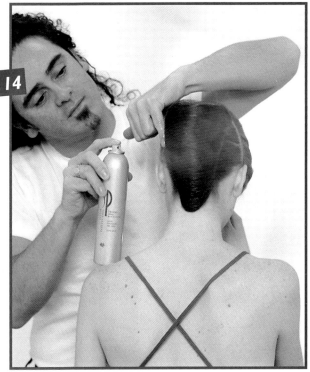

14. Mist with hairspray.

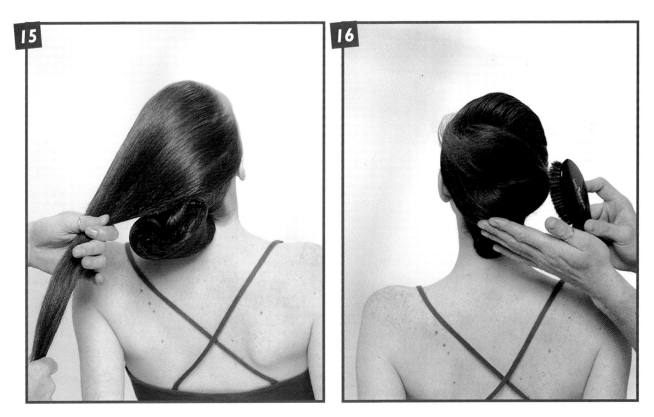

15. Smooth front section backwards and to one side.

16. Twist round top half of pleat and grip. Smooth with brush.

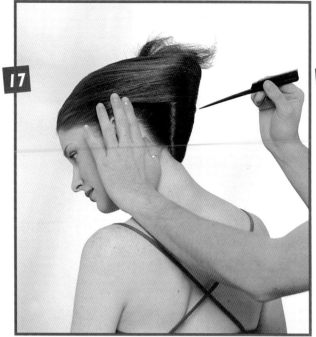

17. Neaten back of pleat using a tailcomb.

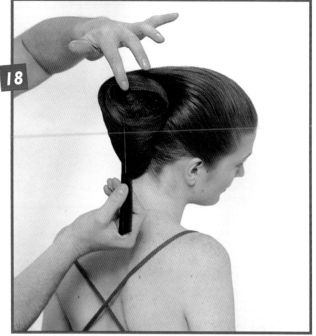

18. Smooth ends in a circular motion to form a curl that follows line at top of pleat. Add sprigs of fresh ivy.

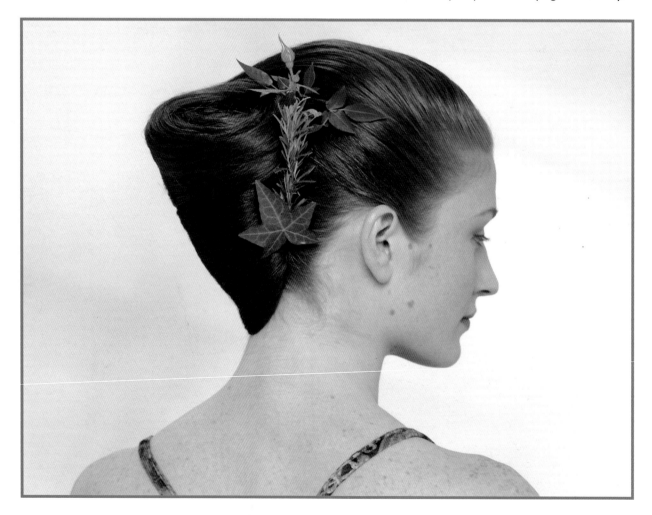

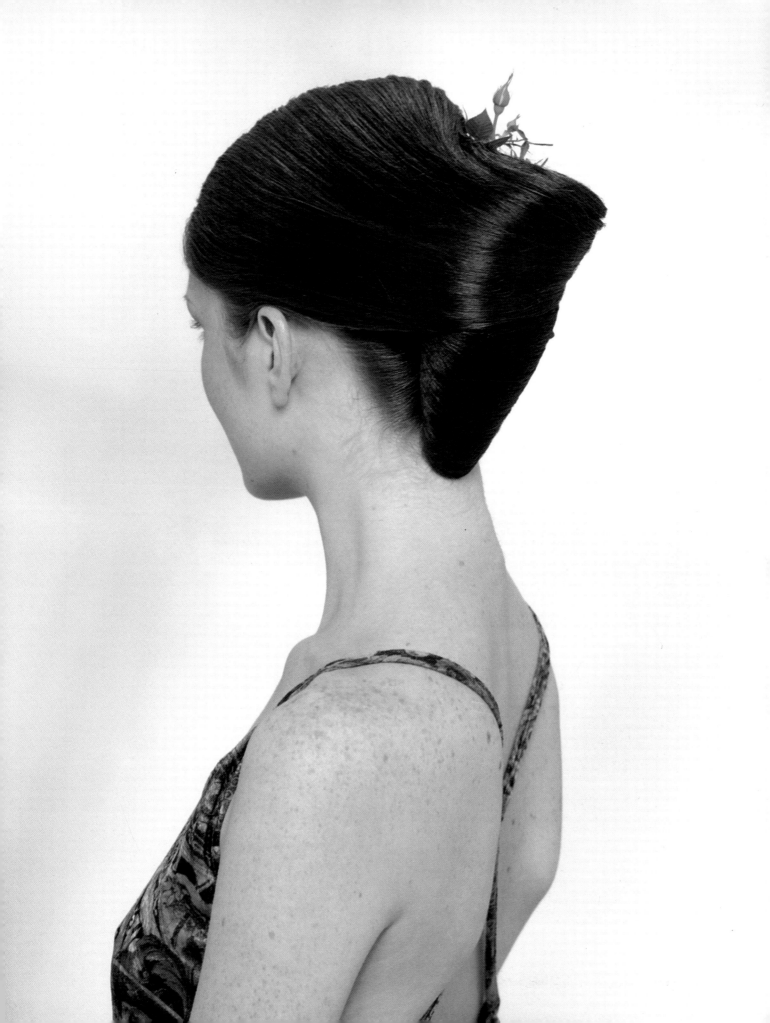

BOUFFANT
Modern version of the classic beehive.

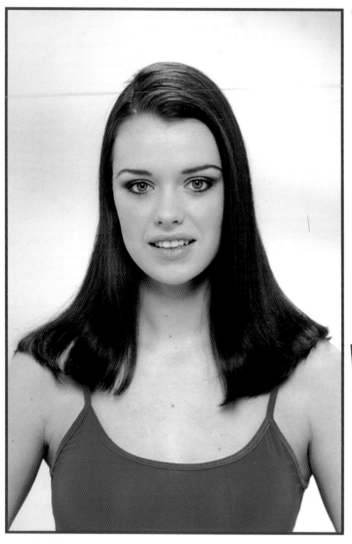

Before

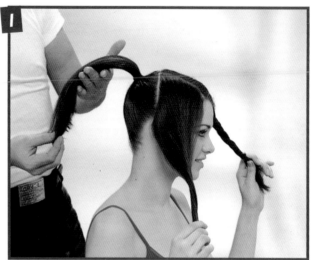

1. Section off front hair from ear to ear. Divide front hair into two sections and put back hair into a high ponytail.

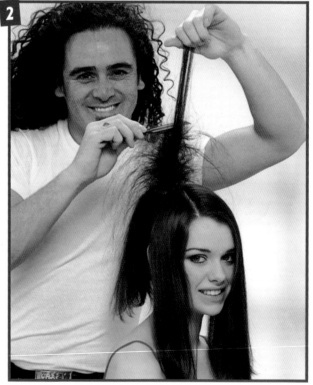

2. Backcomb ponytail.

Tip
When sweeping up side hair always keep tension even. The bouffant can be made smaller by folding the hair more tightly.

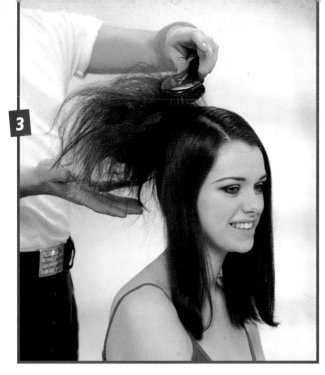

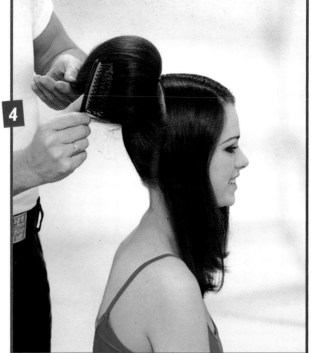

3. Use a bristle brush to begin smoothing top layer of hair only.

4. Gather smoothed ponytail into one hand.

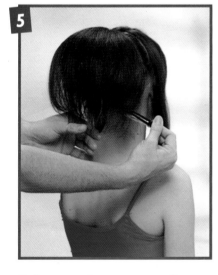

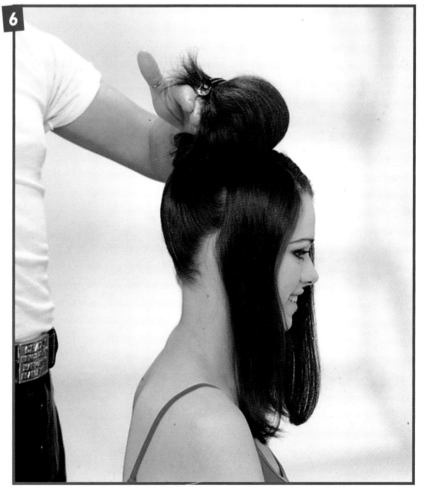

5. Secure ends in a section clip.

6. Flip ponytail forward and grip in a horseshoe shape, 2.5 cm from band.

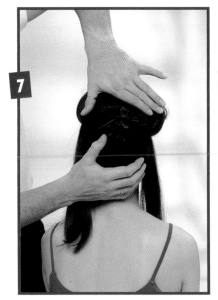

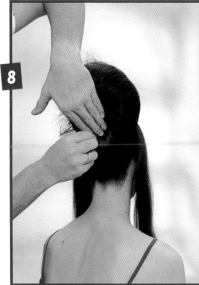

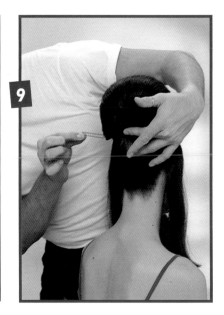

7. Shows grips in place.

8. Flip hair back over and fold round to create a rounded shape. Grip at centre back. Work right side, then left side and lastly top area.

9. Secure sides with hair pins.

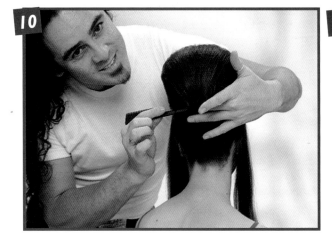

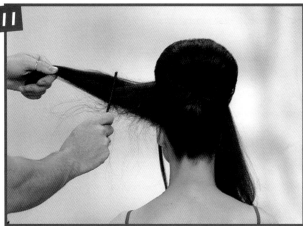

10. Neaten edges with a tailcomb.

11. Backcomb one front section leaving a small band of hair free.

12. Mist with hairspray then smooth this section and pull upwards at a 45° angle so it sweeps around bun.

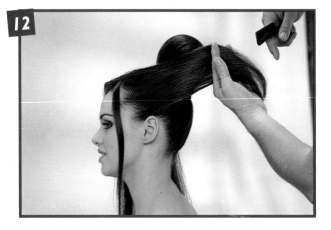

> ❝ Dark hair can be given a lustrous shine by using a longer-lasting semi-permanent colour that adds tone and depth.❞

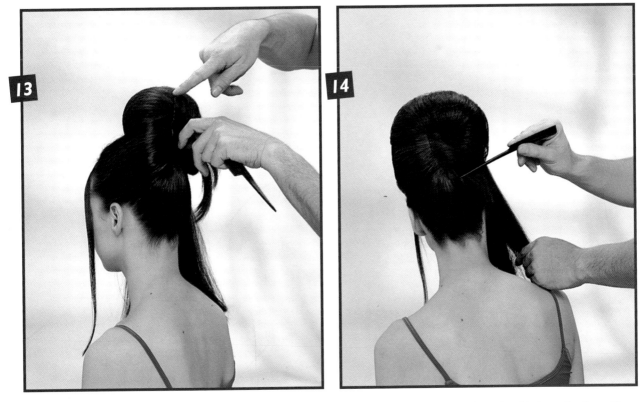

13. Secure, just off centre back, using two hairgrips.

14. Use a tailcomb to tuck ends of hair under bun. Pin to hold in place.

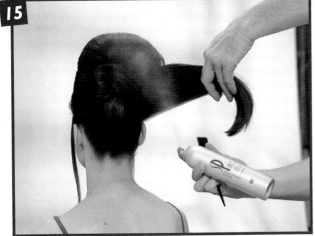

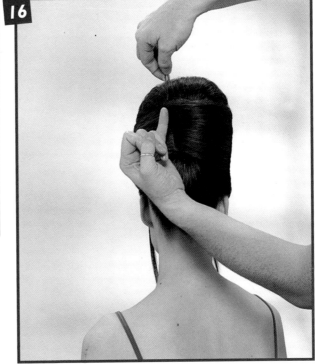

15. Backcomb and mist other side of hair with hairspray. Again leave a small band of hair free as for first side section.

16. Wrap hair round to back and secure with two grips.

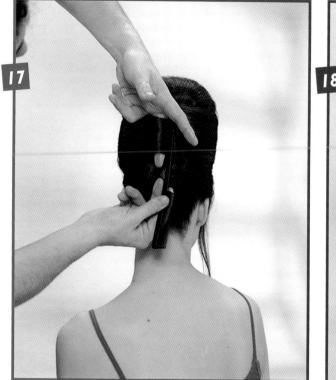

17. Fold ends round finger and form into a barrel curl with tailcomb.

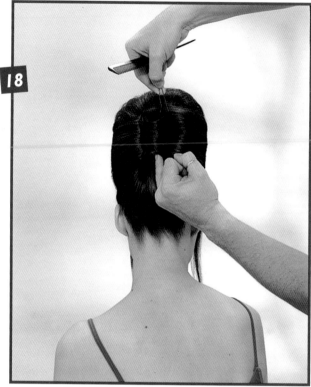

18. Neaten ends and grip in place.

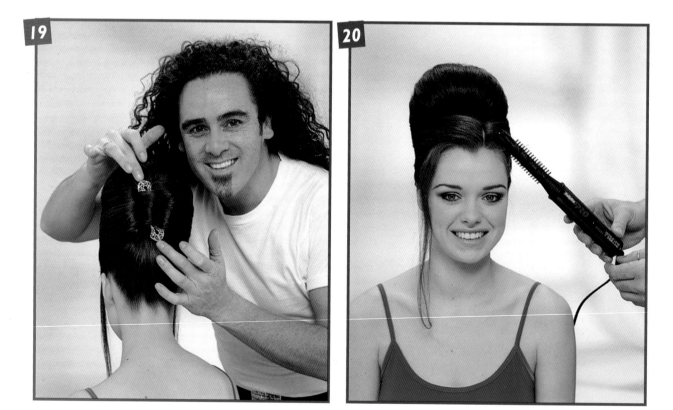

19. Insert hair accessories.

20. Curl side hair into tendrils.

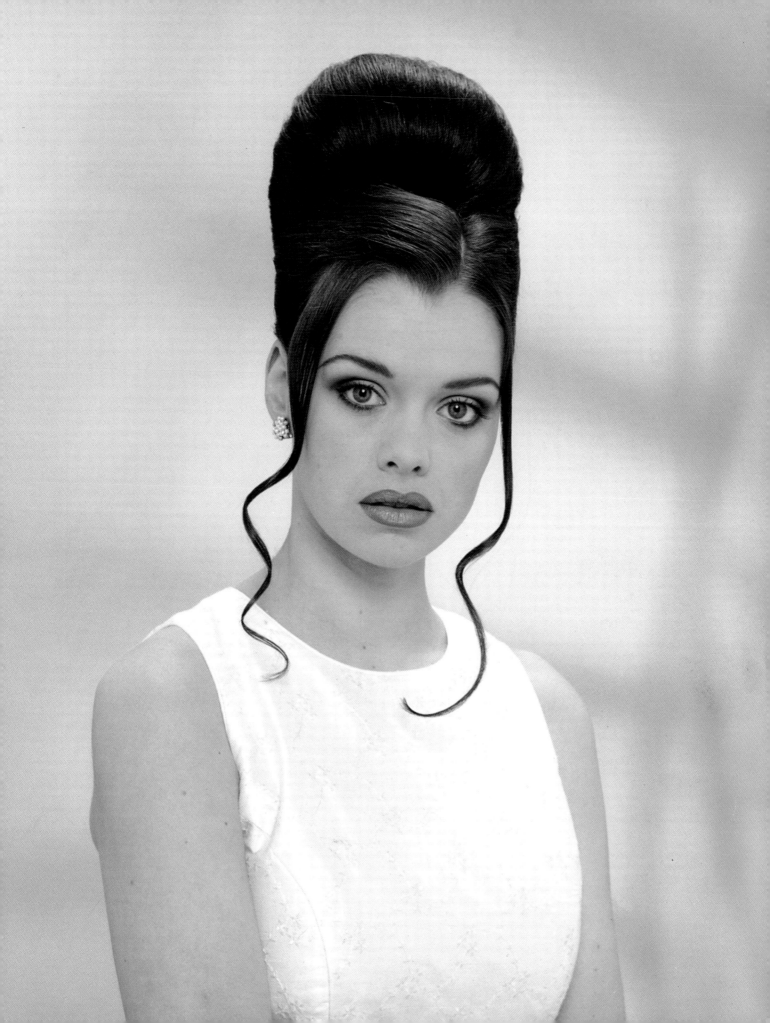

TWIST CHIGNON

A thirties style is given a fresh, modernist look.

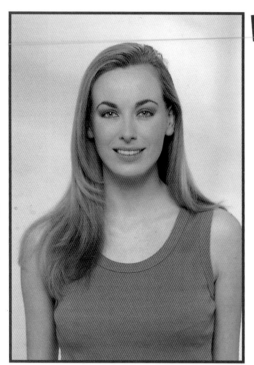

Before

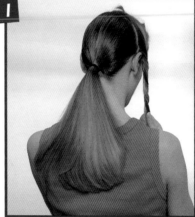

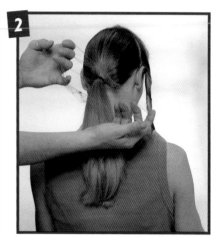

1. Section off front hair from ear to ear and secure back hair in a low ponytail.

2. Fix hairnet to base of ponytail.

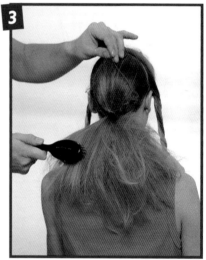

Tip

It is important to decide on placing of flowers or hair accessories before completing the look so they become an integral part of the finished look.

3. Backcomb ponytail, mist with spray and smooth over top layer.

4. Lower hairnet to enclose hair.

5. Set top section of front hair on heated rollers, leaving side sections free.

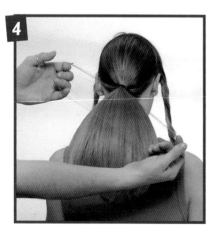

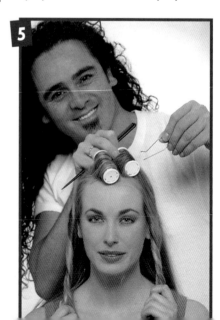

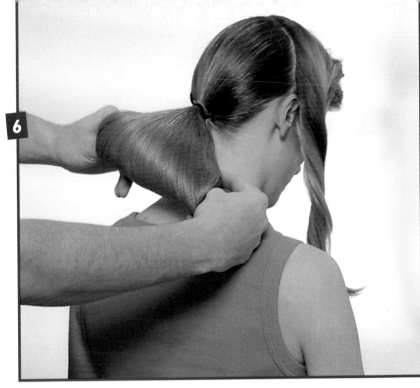

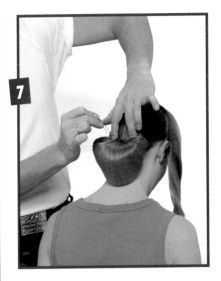

6. Roll under netted ponytail to create a horseshoe shape.

7. Secure with pins.

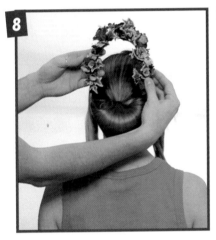

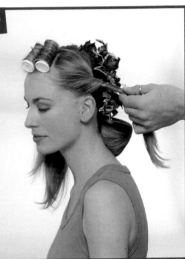

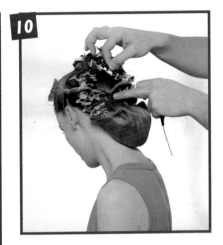

8. Take a garland of flowers, form into a horseshoe shape, roll round and place ends of garland inside ends of roll. Secure with hairgrips.

9. Take one side section of hair and twist in a clockwise direction.

10. Take this section of hair over garland to centre back and secure with pins.

11. Twist end into a curl and repeat with hair at other side.

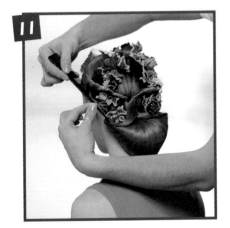

12. Remove heated rollers and backcomb front hair, mist with hairspray and smooth over into a quiff. Hold shape with section clips whilst pinning hair into a coil above head-dress. Mist with hairspray.

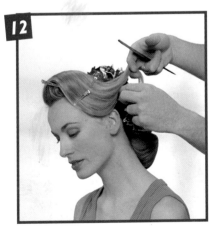

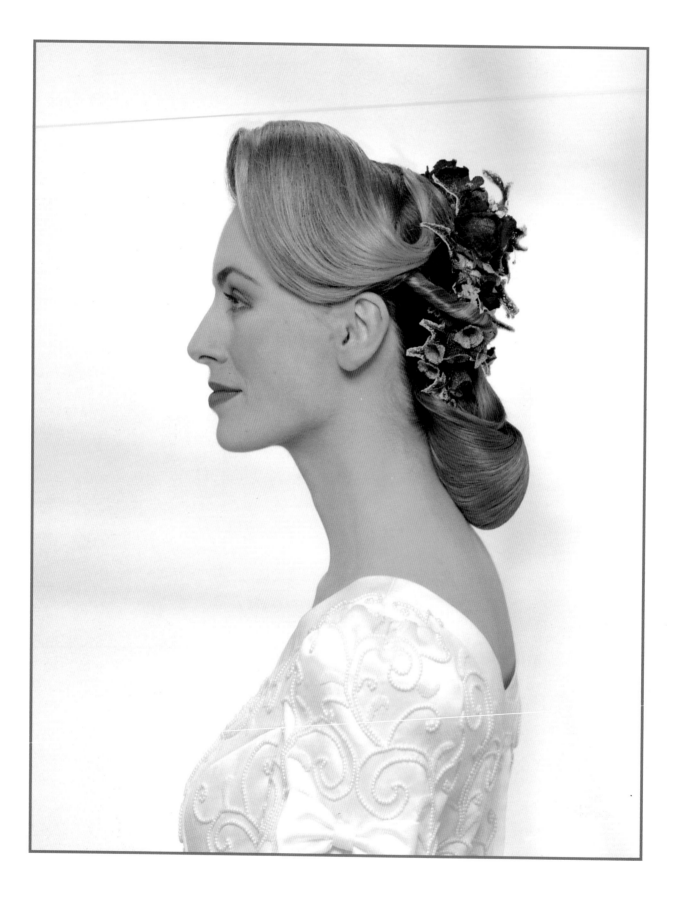

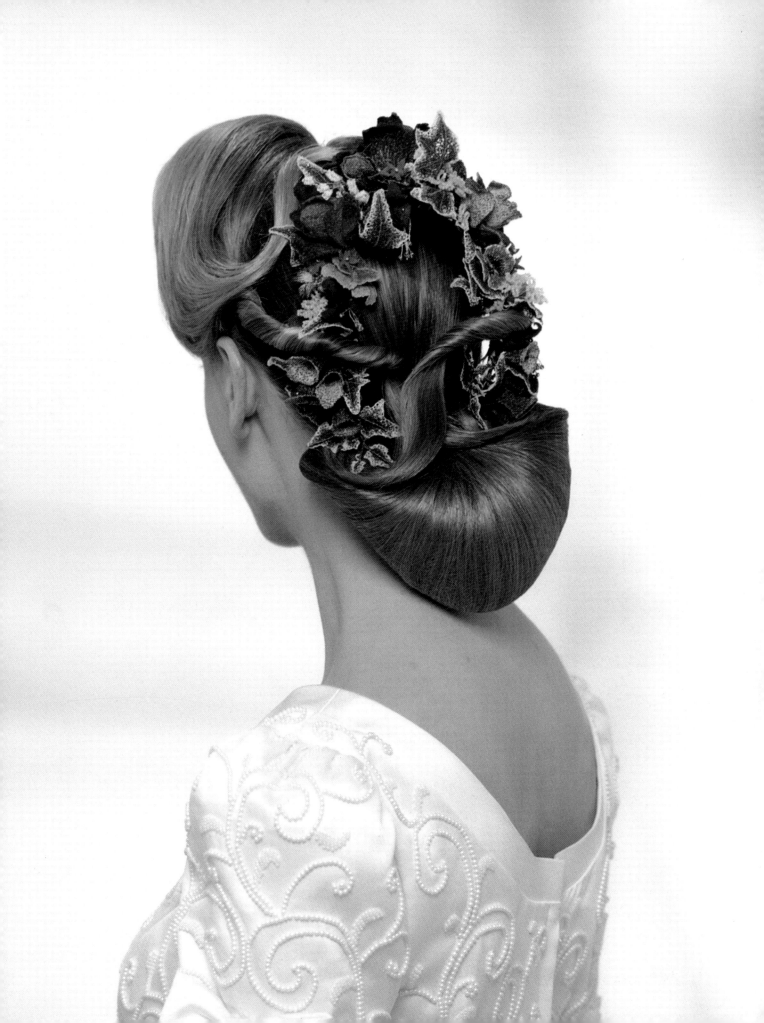

ENTWINED BRAID

Formal braids are softened by balancing with flick-ups.

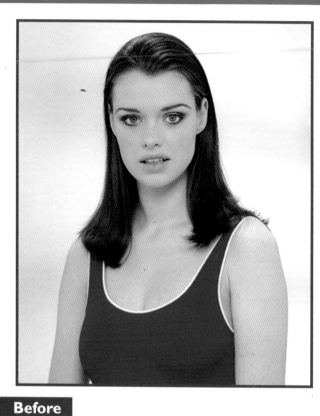

Before

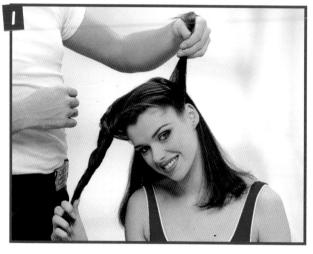

1. Divide off front hair from ear to ear. Take a small section of hair from behind one ear.

Tip

Always work neatly, ensuring partings are straight and accurately defined.

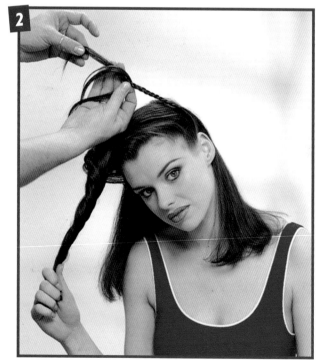

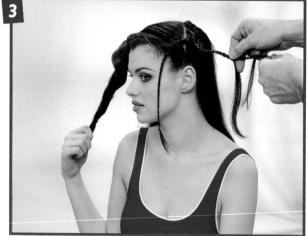

2. Divide this section into three equal amounts and plait upwards. Secure ends of braid with a grip.

3. Moving round, take another small section, plait downwards.

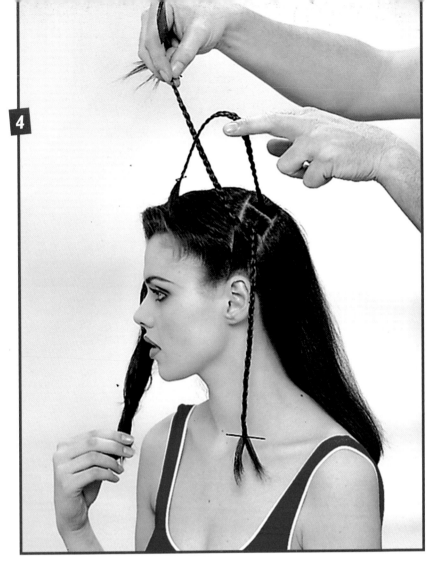

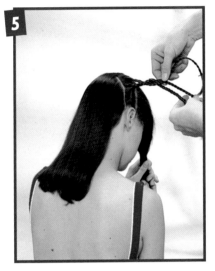

4. Take a third section and plait downwards.

5. Take the three plaits and plait together.

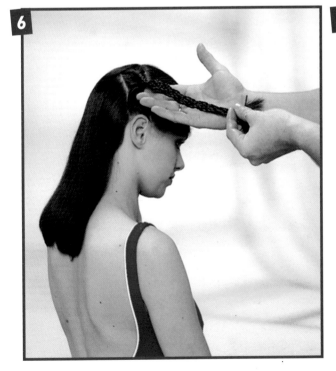

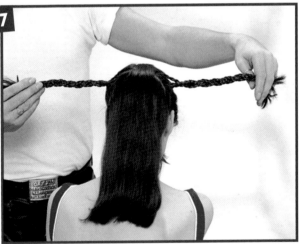

6. Hold ends with a hairgrip. Repeat plaiting process on other side.

7. Shows plaits completed.

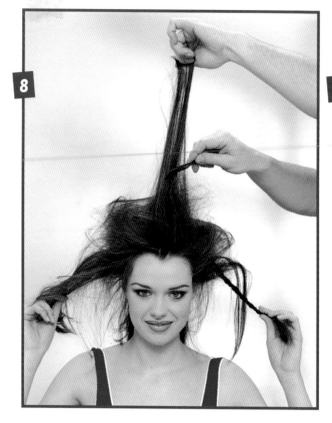 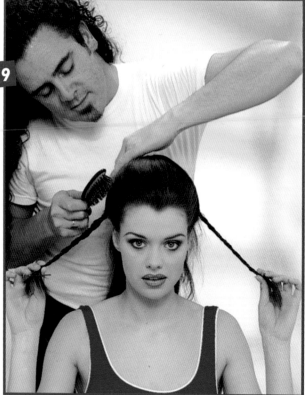

8. Backcomb remaining front hair. Mist with hairspray.

9. Smooth back using a bristle brush and secure into a ponytail.

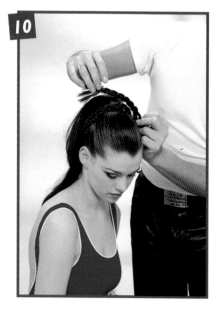 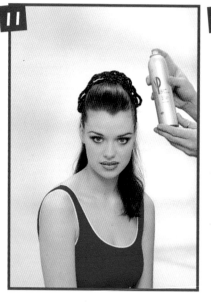 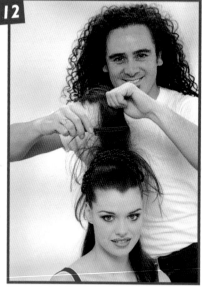

10. Take one plaited section up and over crown and pin in place. Take other plait and place on top of first one to build height. Pin.

11. Mist plaits with hairspray to hold in place.

12. Backcomb ponytail, smooth over and divide into two.

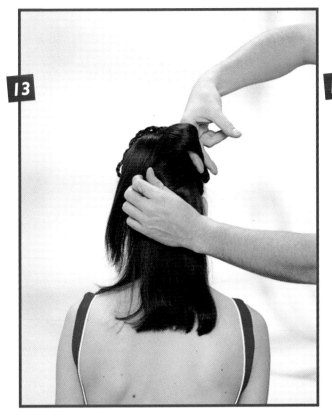

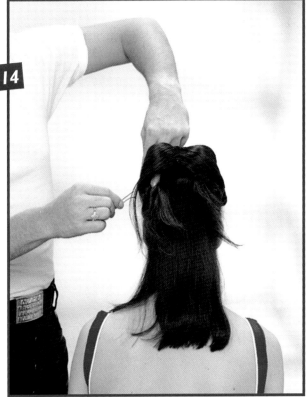

13. Form one half into a barrel curl and pin. Swirl ends of hair up and secure inside barrel curl and pin.

14. Repeat for second half of hair.

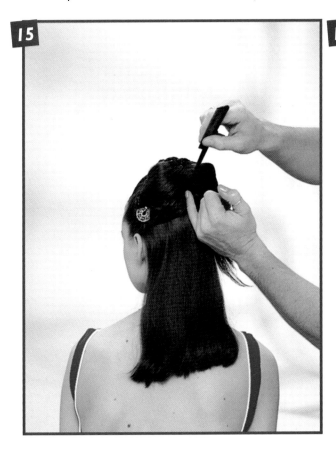

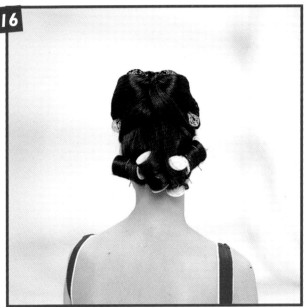

15. Curl ends in using a tailcomb and pin in place. Add hair accessories.

16. Mist lower hair with setting spray and wind onto heated rollers. When rollers are quite cool, remove and brush hair into flick-ups using a bristle brush.

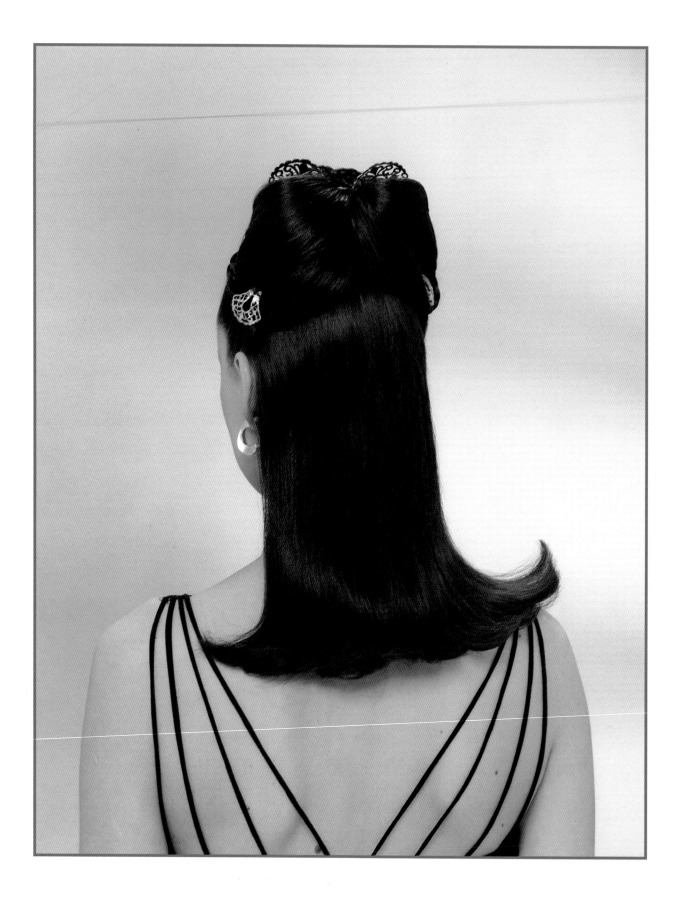

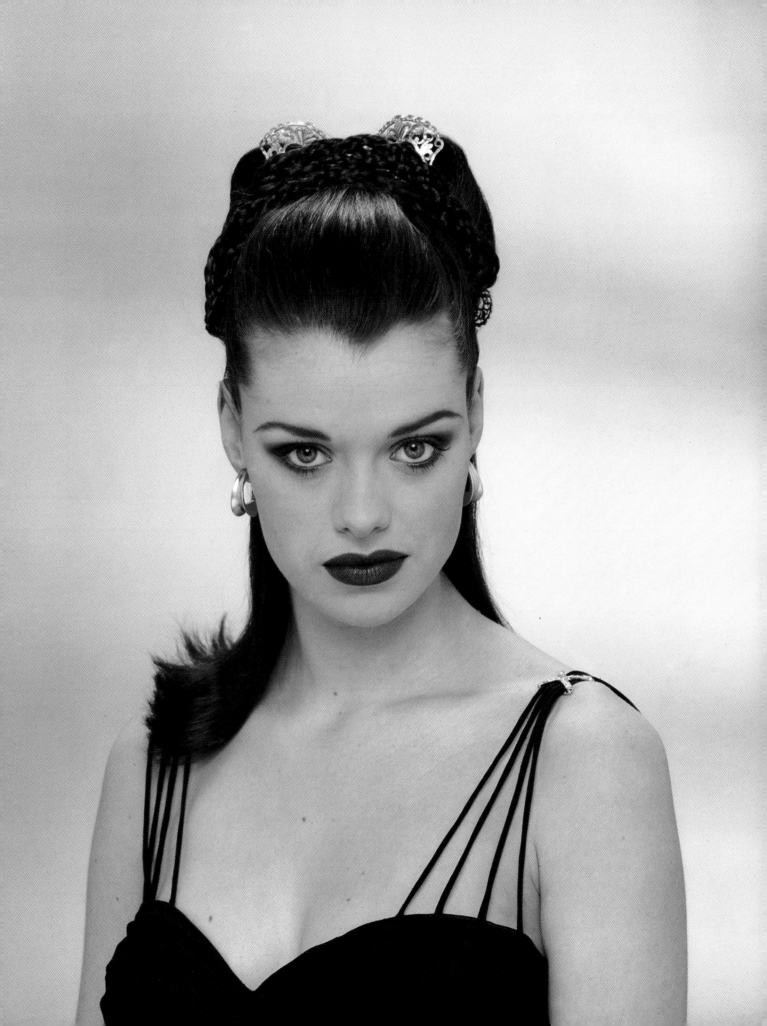

CRESCENT

A rolled bun with an interesting back twist.

Before

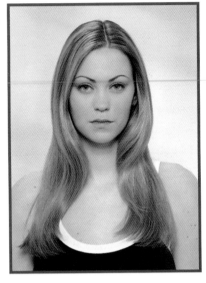

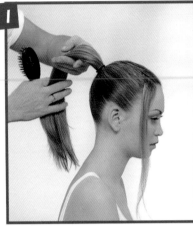

1. Brush hair up into a high ponytail, leaving two small sections at front.

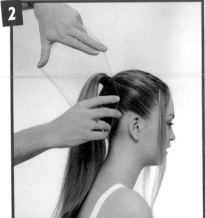

2. Fix a hairnet to base of ponytail.

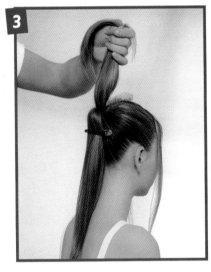

3. Divide ponytail into two equal sections.

4. Backcomb top section then mist with hairspray.

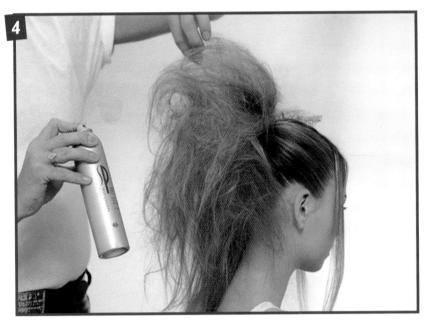

5. Smooth over top layer of this section and pull down net to encase hair.

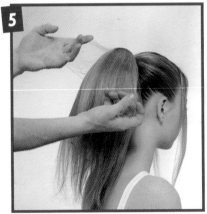

Tip
Be methodical when you work, taking a section of hair at a time and completing before moving on to next section.

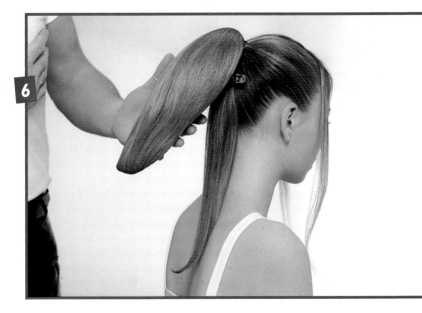

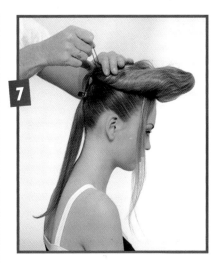

6. Shows top, backcombed ponytail in net. Keep lower ponytail flat with a section clip.

7. Flip netted ponytail over and push a hairpin through, fixing the netted ponytail with a row of crossed grips, 1 cm from base of ponytail in a horseshoe shape.

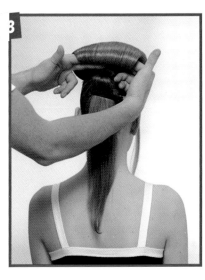

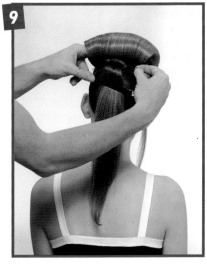

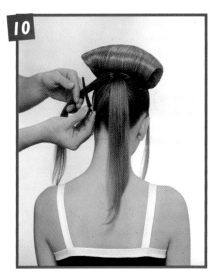

8. Fold ponytail back whilst rolling round fingers.

9. Grip into position on top of other ponytail.

10. Divide lower ponytail into two equal sections and take left-hand section towards front and hold in place with section clip.

11. Fold round sides of roll and pin in position. Repeat for other side.

12. Two tails of hair now remain.

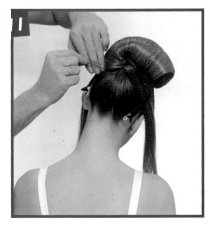

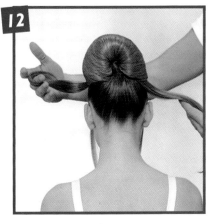

13. Now smooth other tail section round to front, neaten with tailcomb, and pin in place along front of bun.

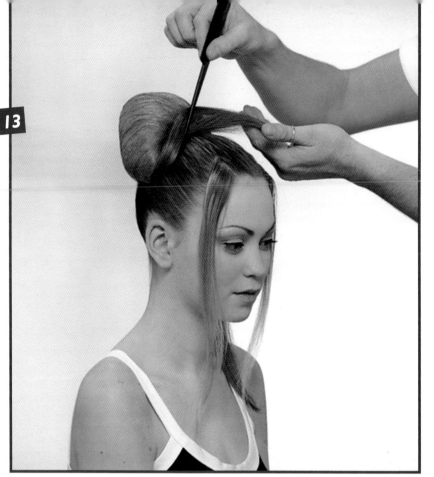

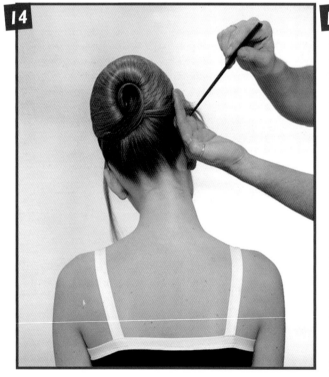

14. Take one tail of hair and form into a curl at centre back of rolled bun. Pin in place, bring the ends of the tail round to front.

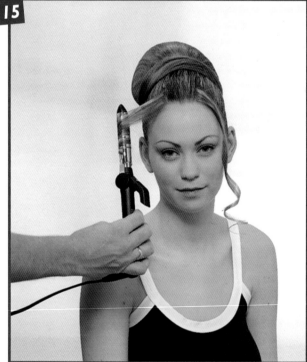

15. Tong side hair to form loose tendrils.

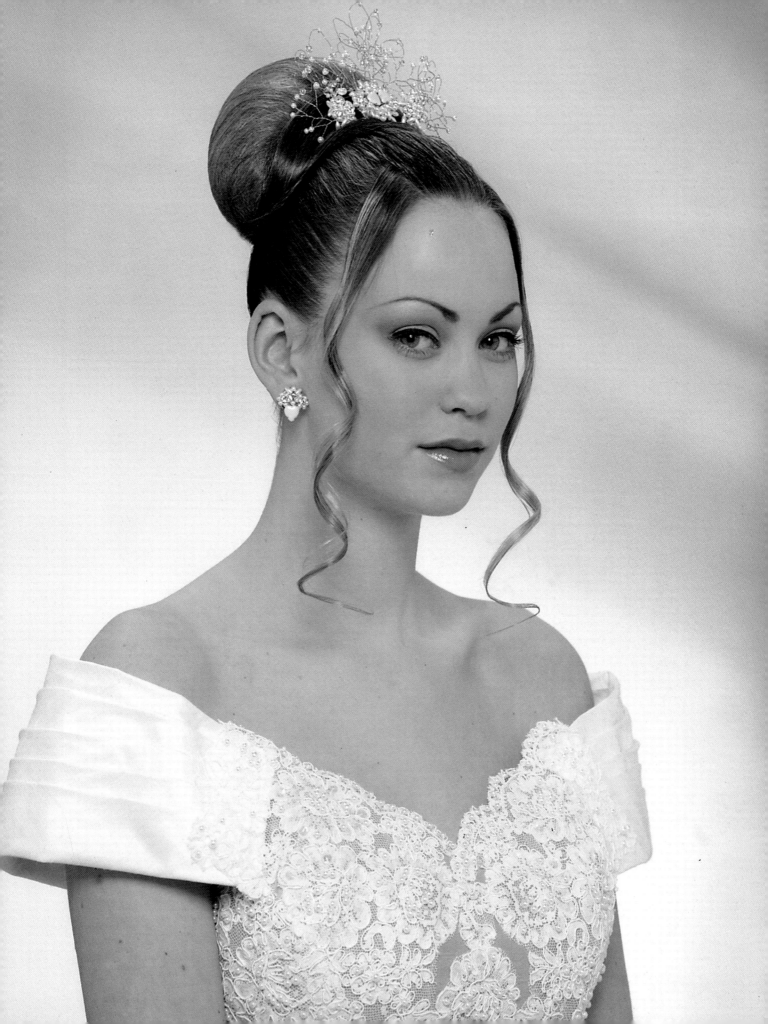

LOOP

Before

1. Take a square section of hair on top of head, leave fringe and a few tendrils at sides free.

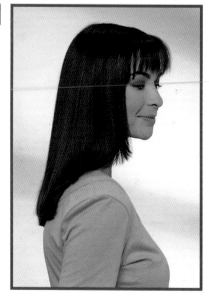

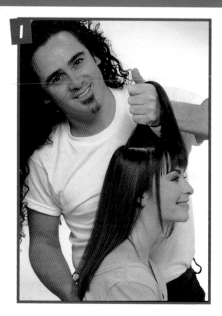

2. Divide off a diagonal section from nape to centre crown and secure in a ponytail.

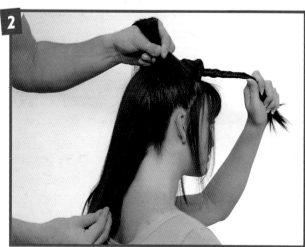

3. Repeat for other side.

4. Take remaining back section of hair and secure in a ponytail.

5. Backcomb each ponytail.

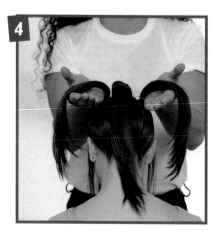

Tip

Balance is all important for this style. Make sure the ponytails are far enough back to allow room to form the style on the top of head.

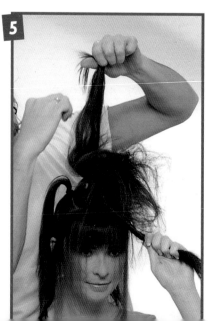

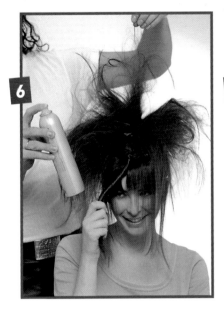

6. Mist with hairspray.

7. Use a bristle brush to smooth top layer of each ponytail and secure ends in a section clip.

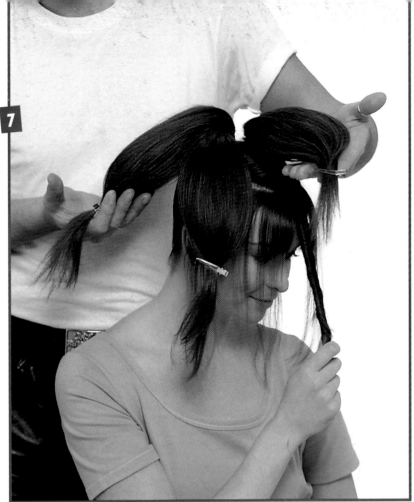

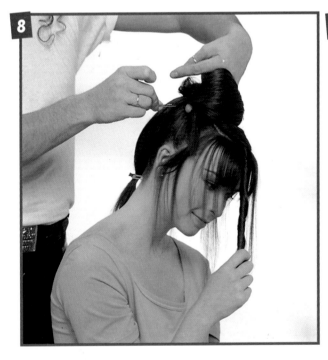

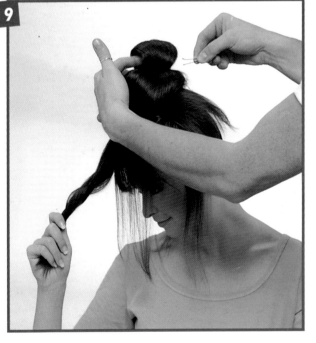

8. Taking one section at a time, twist round hand to form a barrel curl. Grip in place.

9. Take another section and repeat, layering the curls on top of each other and pinning in place as you go. Repeat for third ponytail.

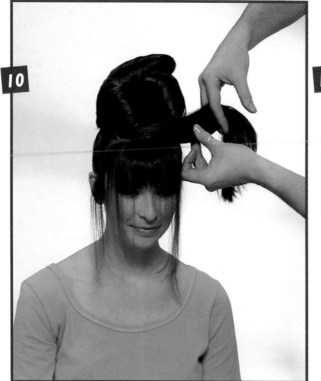

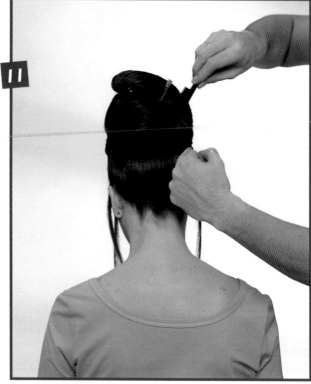

10. Take reserved front section of hair and spread through fingers then loop around the base of curls.

11. Neaten ends using a tailcomb.

12. Form ends into a soft curl and secure with pins.

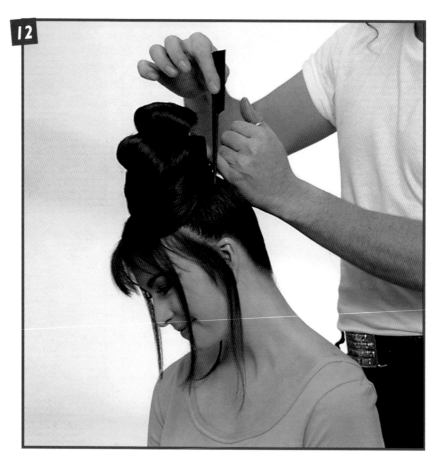

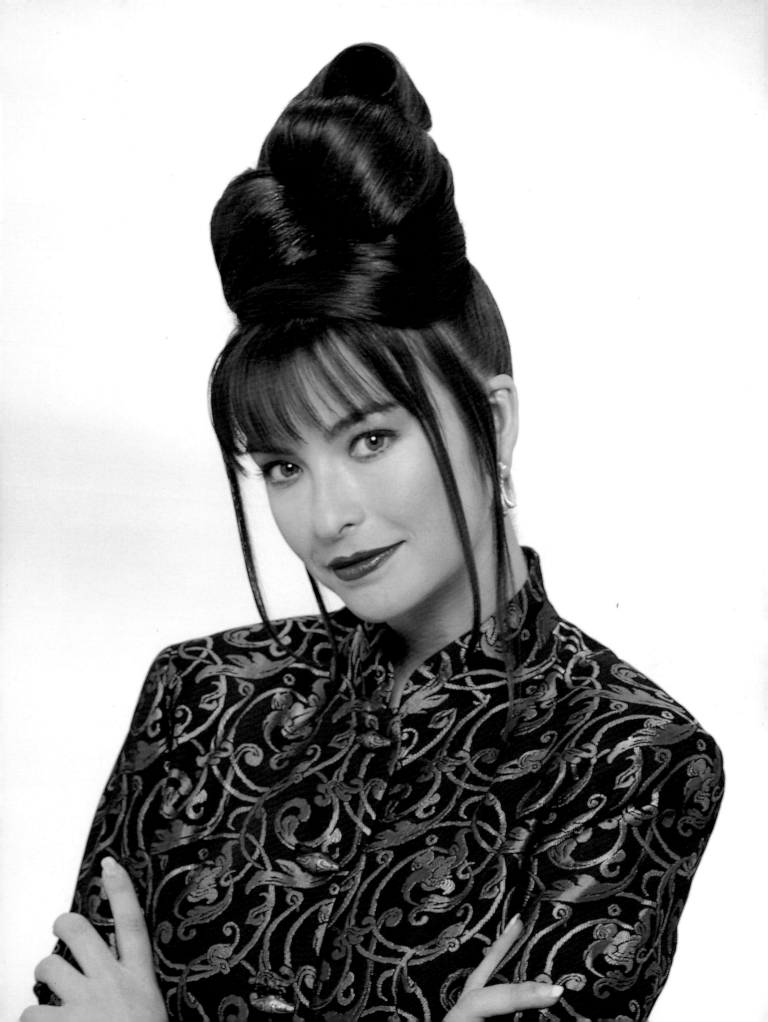

HALO

Before

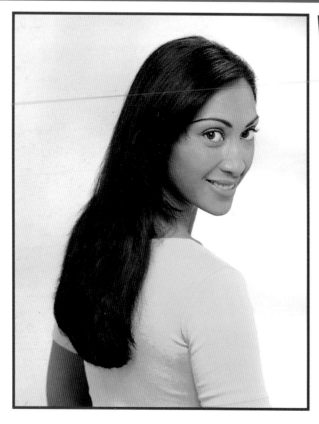

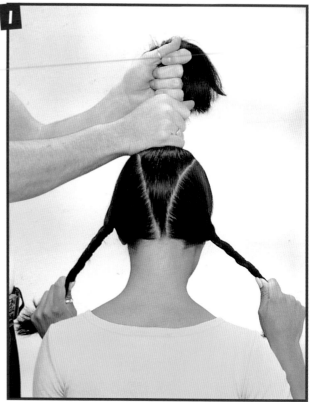

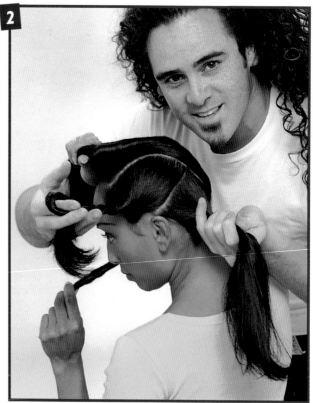

1. Divide off a triangular central section and hold on crown. Twist side hair. This section goes from front to back.

2. Divide one side section into two, and secure lower hair in a ponytail, positioning towards centre back.

Tip

The secret of this style is to keep the top ponytails together so you can create large raised barrel curls which fit loosely together.

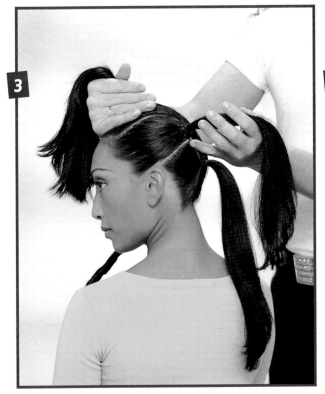

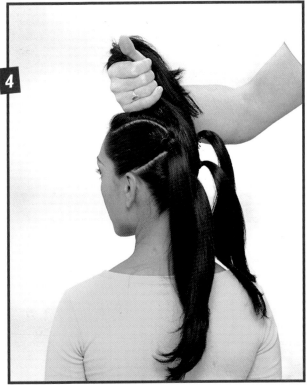

3. Secure top half of this section in a ponytail, positioning towards centre back. Repeat for other side.

4. You now have four ponytails. Take reserved crown hair and brush smooth. Divide off front piece – our model had a long fringe section.

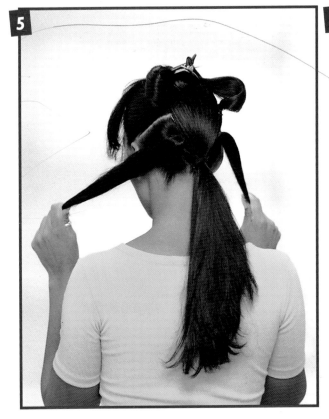

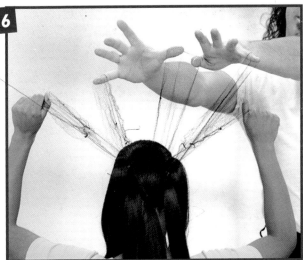

5. Take remaining front hair and brush smooth to centre back of head and secure at nape in a low ponytail. Picture shows this work complete with the two higher ponytails clipped up and out of the way.

6. Grip a net to the base of each ponytail.

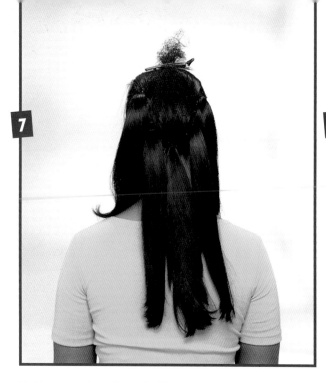

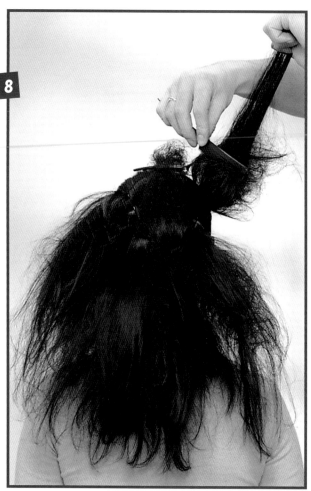

7. Use a section clip to hold nets on crown while you continue to work.

8. Backcomb each ponytail.

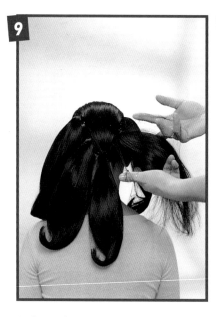

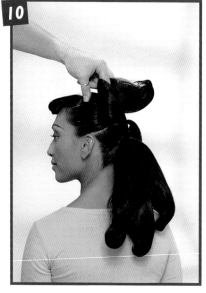

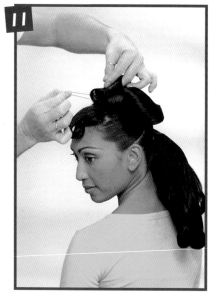

9. Smooth each ponytail and cover with nets, coiling ends into large curls.

10. Coil one section of hair round fingers and grip in place.

11. Coil end over end and pin in place.

12. Repeat with another section.

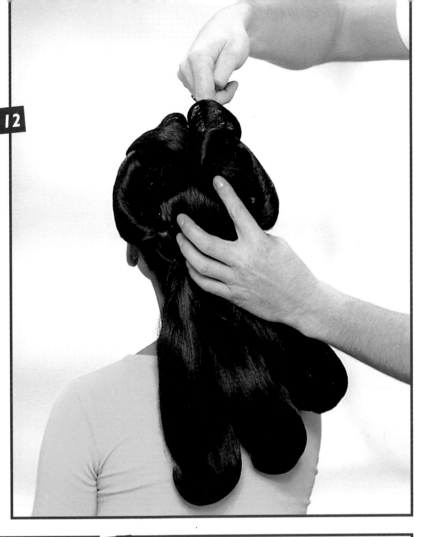

13. Continue in same manner.

14. Use end of tailcomb to tidy curls.

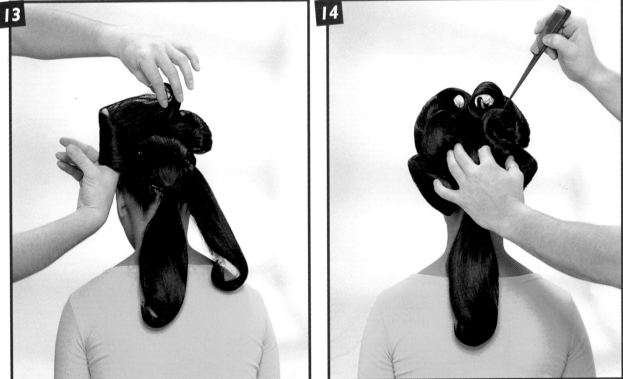

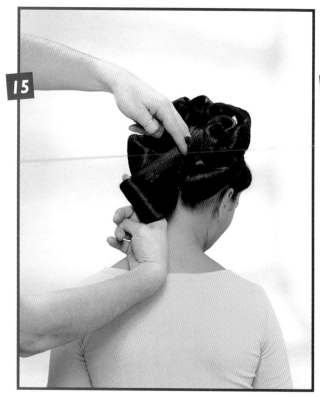

15. Curl final lower ponytail section.

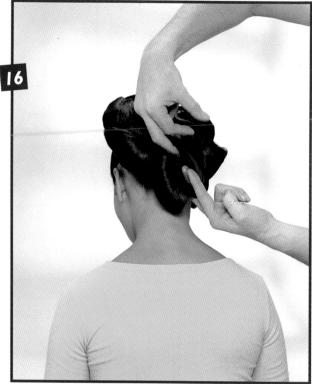

16. Neaten ends and pin.

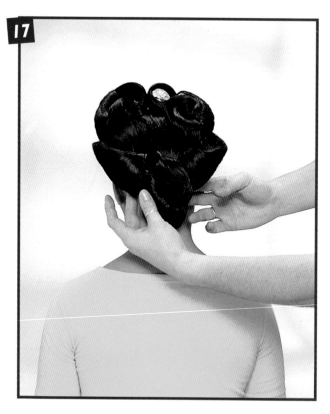

17. Shows completed back of style before addition of flowers.

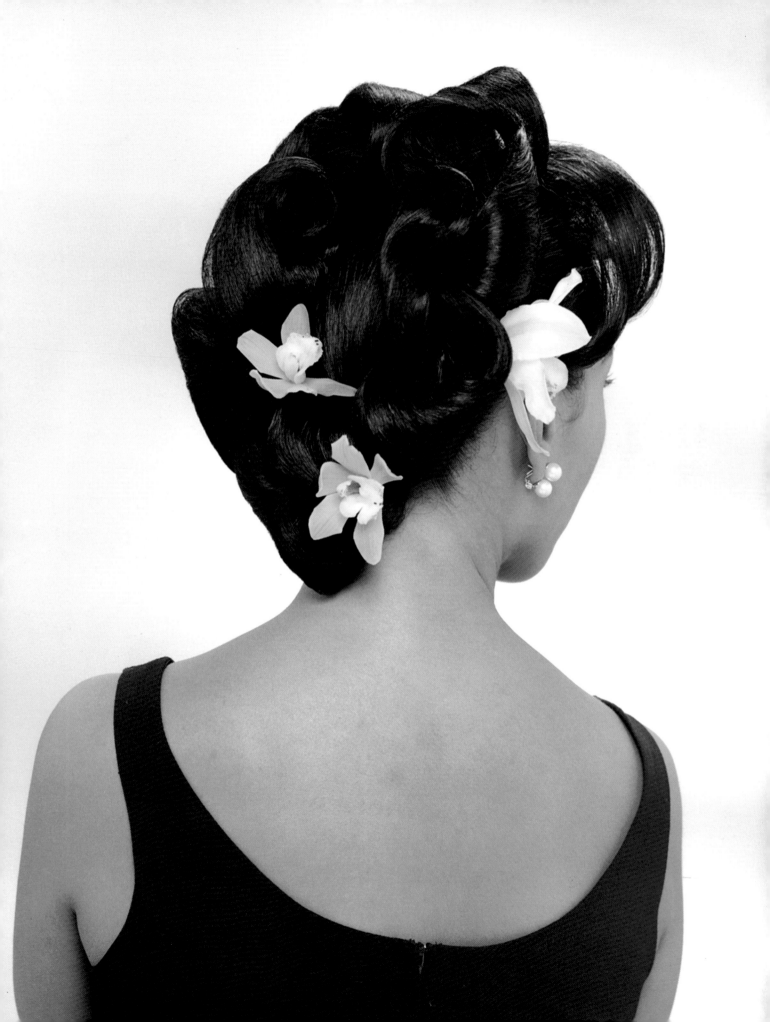

SCULPT

Swirls combine with formed curls to give a beautiful textural mix.

Before

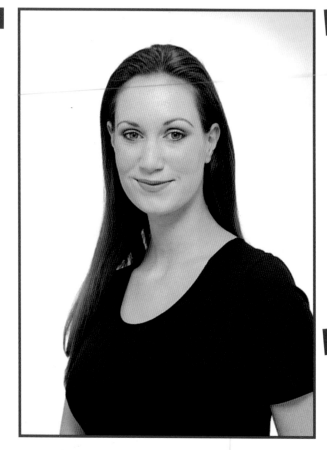

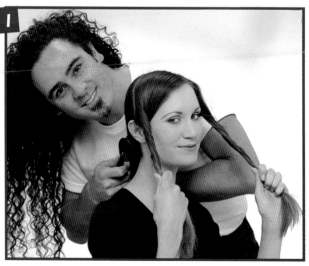

1. Section off front hair from ear to ear. Divide front hair into two sections and smooth back hair down.

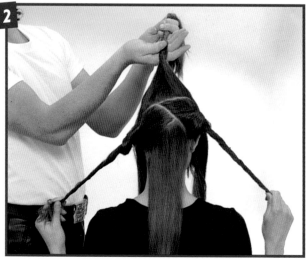

2. Divide back hair diagonally into four sections.

3. Clasp each of these four sections into a ponytail. It is important that the ponytails are close together — they should be able to sit inside clasped hands — see picture.

Tip

This style works best if the ponytails are positioned close together and each is worked flat like a ribbon so the sculpting of each curl is easier.

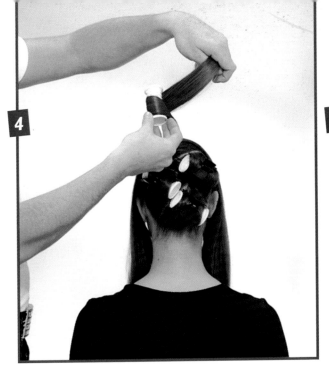

4. Mist ponytails with setting lotion and set on heated rollers, leave to cool and remove.

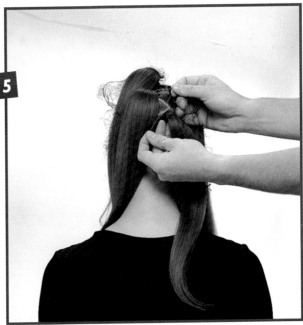

5. Use a grip to attach a hairnet to the base of each ponytail.

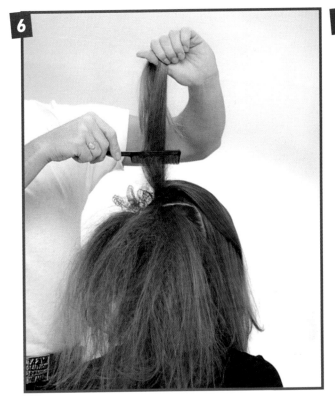

6. Backcomb each ponytail

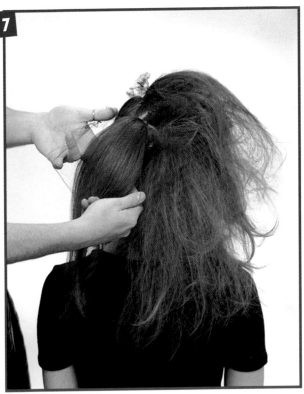

7. Use a bristle brush to smooth over top layer of one ponytail then enclose in hairnet. Repeat for other ponytails.

8. Mist with hairspray.

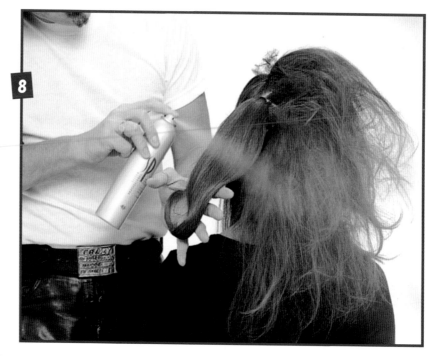

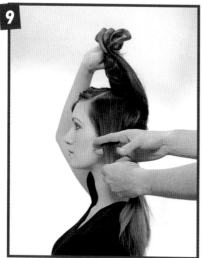

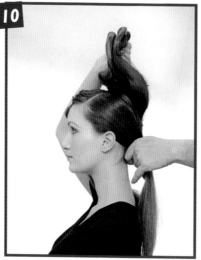

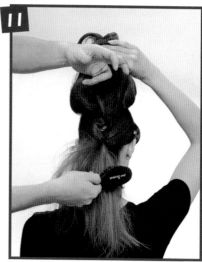

9. Lift netted hair up and smooth front sections back.

10. Take front sections of hair and secure at centre back in a ponytail.

11. Backcomb and smooth the back ponytail.

12. Attach hairnet to base of back ponytail.

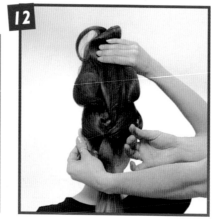

"Wear and tear on hair can be minimised by adopting a hair-care regime that includes regular cutting, shampooing and conditioning, combined with the daily use of high-quality styling products and equipment. **"**

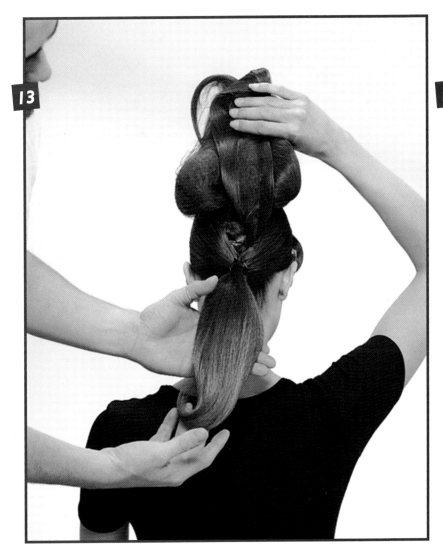

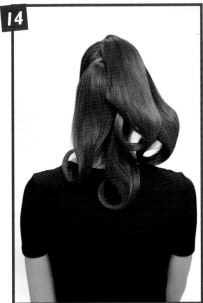

13. Enclose back ponytail in a hair-net. Mist with hairspray.

14. Shows completed netted hair.

15. Take top ponytail and using two fingers coil into a barrel curl.

16. Grip in place.

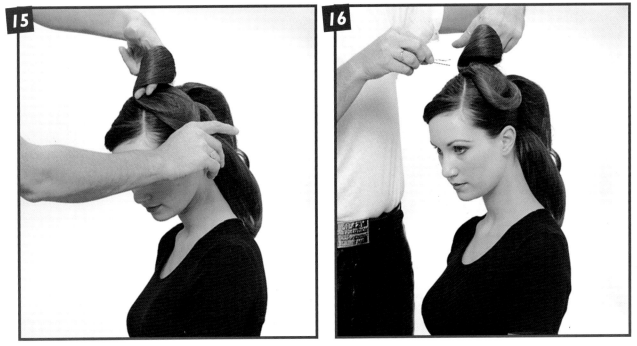

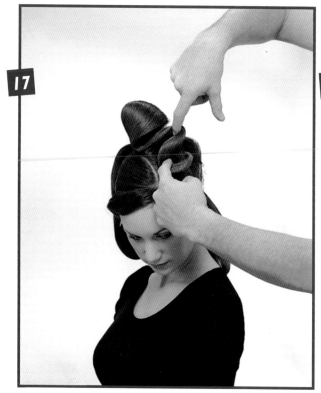

17. Form end into an S shape and pin.

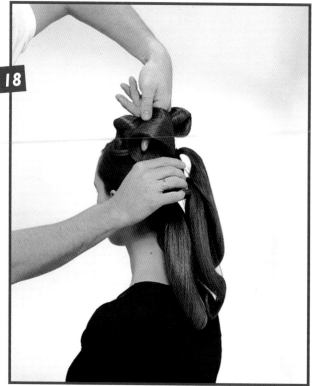

18. Repeat with next ponytail.

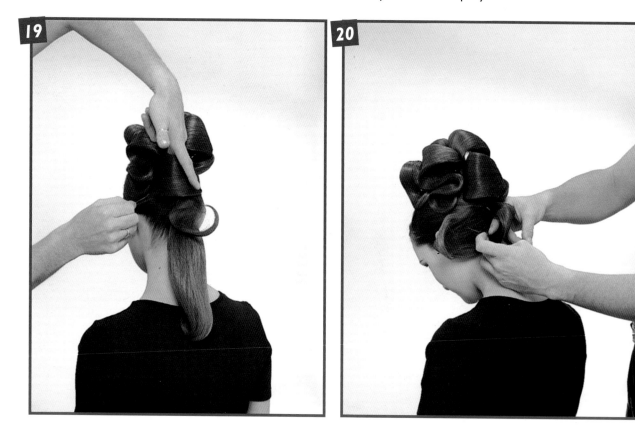

19. Continue working in same manner, curling, pinning and twisting.

20. Position and pin final curl.

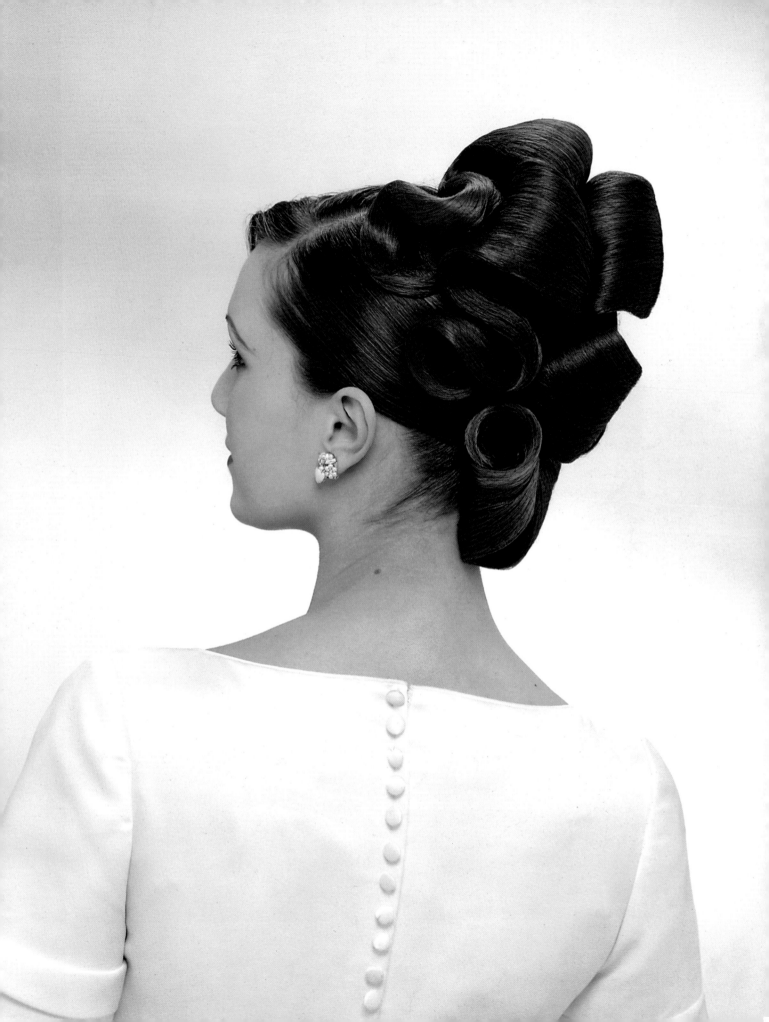

PART 3

EQUIPMENT AND

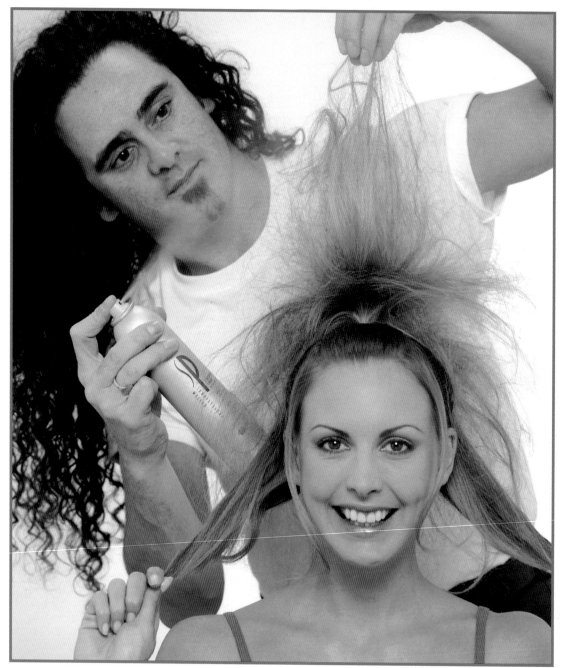

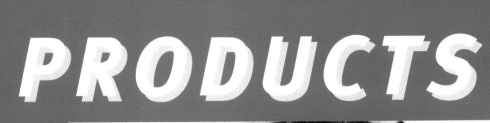

PRODUCTS

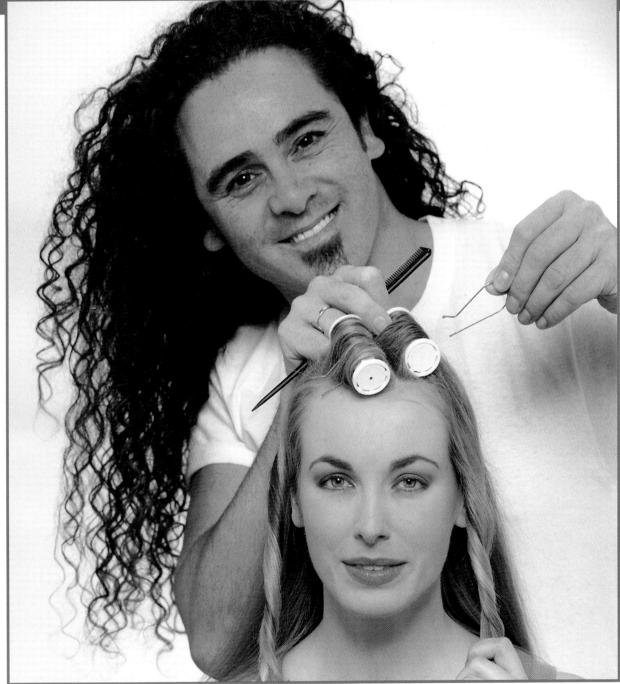

BRUSHES, COMBS...

*T*he right tools not only make hairdressing more fun but also make styling much easier. Invest in high-quality equipment that is kind to hair and scalp. Choose from one of the professional ranges, such as Denman, which has been manufactured in the United Kingdom since 1938 and has developed a worldwide reputation for exceptional standards of quality, performance and durability. Denman products are exported to more than 50 countries, and the Denman philosophy is to provide hair designers, their clients and the general public with a comprehensive range of quality styling brushes and accessories to help achieve the best styling results time after time.

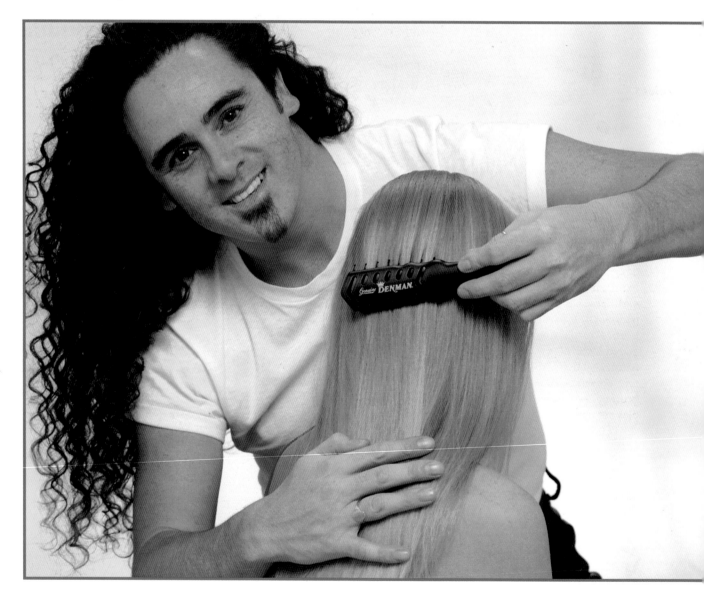

AND SELF-FIXING ROLLERS

Radial or **round brushes** are used to create volume and curl. They can also be used to straighten hair and to control naturally curly or wavy hair whilst blow-drying. Choose flexible-bristle radials for extra grip and control, nylon round brushes for small to medium curls, mixed-bristle 'bottle' brushes for curling, and wooden brushes with mixed bristle in small, medium, large and extra-large for blow-drying.

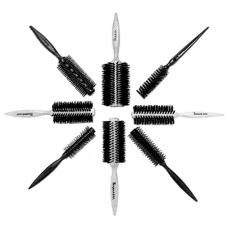

Half-round styling brushes and volume brushes are similar in design. The traditional style offers excellent grip and control and is ideal for smoothing, shaping and polishing the hair. This type of brush incorporates smooth, round-ended nylon pins set into anti-static, natural rubber pads which will not tear or damage the hair. Volume brushes are similar again, with nylon pins set into anti-static rubber pads.

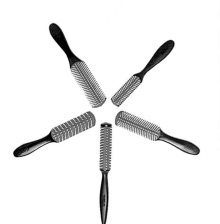

However, the volume brushes have widely spaced pin formations which increase air circulation at root level enabling you to add volume and movement to the hair during blow-drying for a softer, fuller look.

Vent brushes are ideal for disentangling wet or dry hair and are suitable for all hair lengths and types. Widely-spaced pins and vented design allow warm air to circulate directly at root level, accelerating the blow-drying process. Choose tunnel vent for fast blow-drying or Hyflex vent for fast and gentle blowing.

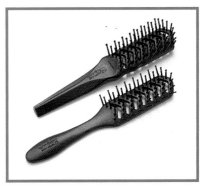

Cushion/flat bristle brushes are the traditional 'dressing table' brush used for grooming and conditioning the hair. Perfect for longer hair, they give smoothness, sheen and reduce static electricity. Choose wild-boar bristle, natural bristle with nylon quill or nylon bristle in small, medium or large sizes.

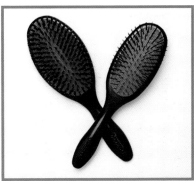

Combs should have saw-cut teeth, which means there are no sharp edges. Use wide-toothed combs for disentangling and combing conditioner through the hair, fine tail-combs for sectioning, and styling combs for grooming.

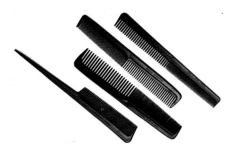

Velcro rollers, which come in many sizes, are perfect for creating curl in wet or dry hair. Quick and easy to use, they need neither clips nor pins.

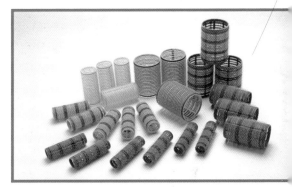

DENMAN — BRITISH MADE. Preferred by Professionals

Denroy International Ltd, Clandeboye Road, Bangor, Co. Down, BT20 3JH, Northern Ireland. Tel.: 01247 462141. Freephone: 0800 262509. Fax: 01247 451654. Export office: 16 Princetown Mews, 167–169 London Road, Kingston upon Thames, Surrey, KT2 6PT, UK. Tel.: 0181 974 6674. Fax: 0181 974 5966.

HEATED STYLING APPLIANCES

Hi-tech electrical styling appliances allow you to dry, curl and straighten hair efficiently. Invest in professional equipment that has been designed in conjunction with hairdressers to give the best possible results.

For example, a salon dryer will have a powerful long-life, heavy-duty, AC motor which is designed for constant use (usually calculated at three full hours a day). Nozzles are slim, which means air comes out with more velocity – making precision drying easier. Consumer models have less powerful, smaller, DC motors, with a fraction of the air thrust. With professional dryers, the strong air thrust gives faster results because hot air streams along the wet hair strand, vibrating and separating. Professional dryers also give 'cold' air blast for finishing. This is not possible on consumer models because the wiring for most DC domestic-type dryers takes the mains power through the element to the motor (the element must always be working to power the motor). The 'cold' shot buttons then modify 'hot' to 'warm' rather than 'cold'.

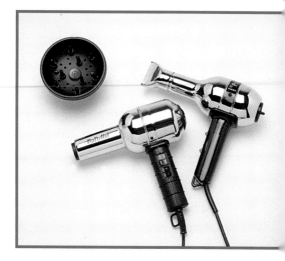

Mille is a chrome-bodied, traditional-style professional dryer made in Italy. A classic tool, it is robust, but with an ultra-slim precision barrel. It has six heat/speed settings, including cold, a removable dual filter, long cord and plastic concentrator nozzle.

Chrome Salon Professional Dryer comes with six heat/speed settings including cold. Complete with concentrator nozzle, diffuser attachment and long cord.

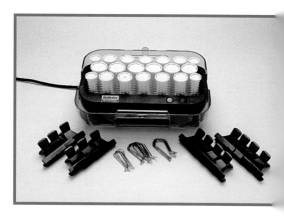

Professional Rollers have cool rims and a concave shape to fit closer to the scalp and give more root lift. The roller set heats up fast and comes with three sizes of roller, fixing pins plus butterfly clamps.

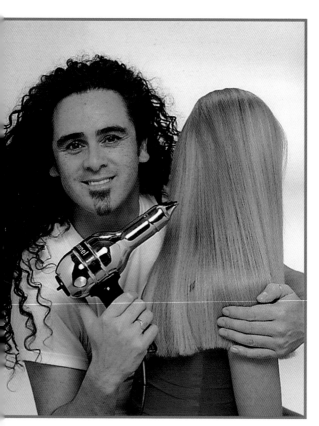

*T*ongs consist of a barrel or prong and a depressor groove. The barrel is round, the depressor is curved to fit around the barrel when the tong is closed. The thickness of the barrel varies, and the size of the tong that is used depends on whether small, medium or large curls are required.

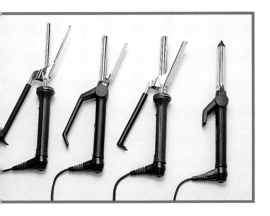

Pro Spring Tongs have a spring-lever form for simple tonging. High temperature only, the barrel is polished and has a cool tip. Available in 13 mm, 16 mm and 19 mm barrel sizes with heat stand.

Original Tongs are slim with a polished chrome barrel and perfect balance and accuracy. Available with heat stand, professional swivel, replaceable cord and on–off switch with light. Available in 13 mm and 18 mm barrel sizes.

Pro Marcel Tongs have an ultra-modern ergonomic design with adjustable tensioning of the clip for loose or tight tonging. The barrel is polished with rounded hot ends for ultra-smooth finish. With two temperatures, it comes with a pro-fessional, replaceable cord and heat stand. Available in 13 mm, 16 mm and 19 mm barrel sizes.

Micro Tongs are ultra slim for tiny curls and ringlets. Polished chrome barrel, heat stand and professional swivel, replaceable cord. On–off switch and light in 9 mm barrel size only.

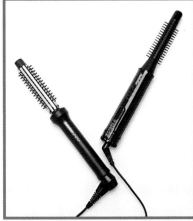

Pro Heat Styling Brushes have ergonomic handle design for easy use. Slightly soft combs for comfort. Professional, retractable cord and heat stand. Available in 13 mm, 16 mm and 19 mm barrel sizes.

Magic Styl'Air is a classic hot-air brush with soft retractable combs. Ready instantly, it is ideal for gentle styling.

Spiral Tongs are the easy way to do ringlets and tiny curls. The barrel is grooved so that hair is perfectly spaced for accurate ringlets. Polished gold barrel with on–off switch and light. Professional swivel, and replaceable cord in 13 mm barrel size.

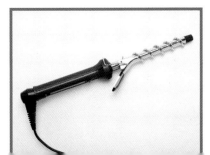

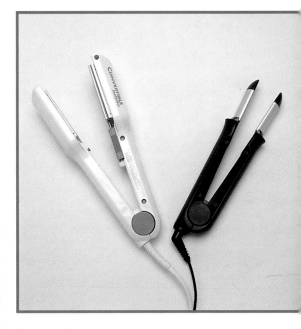

Convertible is a straightener and crimper all in one, with an instant converter switch. High temperature for fast working and anti-stick plates.

Designer is the session stylists' specialist tool that has ultra-slim styling plates to straighten, shape and add texture to the hair. Light, with cool ends for working close to the scalp.

BaByliss

BaByliss

BaByliss (UK) Ltd, Prospect House, Archipelago, Lyon Way, Frimley, Surrey, GU16 5ER, UK. Tel.: 0990 133191. Fax: 01276 687528.

IT'S THE SYSTEM

Wella System Professional is a diagnostic range of integrated products that offers the ultimate hair-care fitness regime for salon and home use. Organically based, highly effective ingredients are delivered via liposomes and hydrobeads for maximum efficacy. The range uses nature-identical preservatives, is biologically degradable, has a skin-friendly pH and has been dermatologically tested. Formulations contain UV filters to protect against environmental assaults, and shine-enhancers to give hair a natural, silky shimmer.

Hair-care prescriptions include treatments, shampoos, conditioners and styling products that work in synergy to create and maintain lustrous, healthy, fit hair.

At the salon, initial treatment includes an aromatherapy head massage that harnesses the healing and regenerative powers of essential oils. This serves to stimulate the circulation whilst developing the effectiveness of the active ingredients in the products used. The massage can be relaxing or invigorating depending on which Massage Complex is selected. Treatment is maintained with home-use products that have been developed to further resolve hair-care problems, repair, regenerate and add a wondrous shine and gloss.

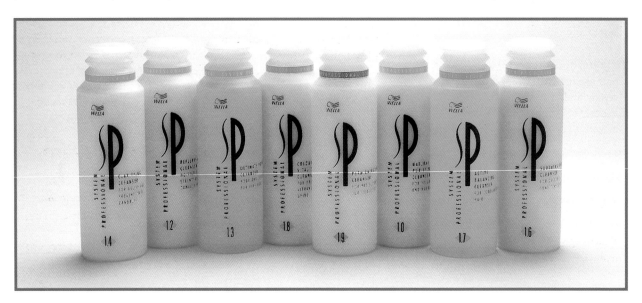

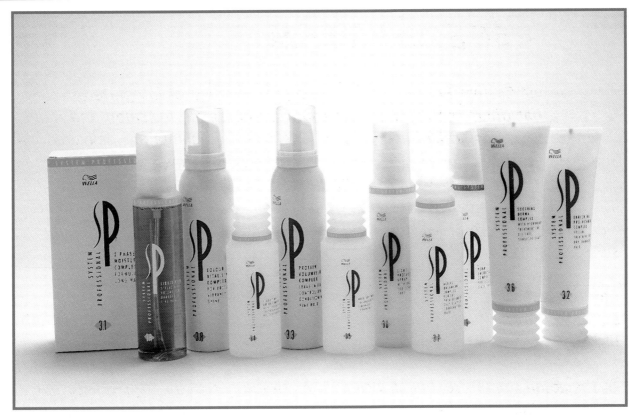

NORMAL AND FREQUENT USE

Natural Purifying Cleanser
Thorough but gentle enough for everyday use, it strengthens and combats static whilst adding vitality and shine.

Light Protection Spray Guards hair against the drying effect of heat styling and UV rays whilst further protecting against trauma from brushing and combing.

LONG

Replenishing Cleanser Levels out the porosity along each hair shaft to give elasticity and vitality, making hair supple and resilient.

2-Phase Moisturising Complex
Adds a protective coating to the hair that effectively strengthens whilst adding shine and suppleness.

DRY AND DAMAGED

Enriching Pro-Vitamin Complex Conditioning boost that strengthens and protects, making hair supple and smooth whilst improving elasticity.

Replenishing Cleanser See under 'Long' on this page.

FINE

Ultimate Volume Cleanser
Herbal acids strengthen hair from the inside while volumisers give body and vitality.

Protein Volumising Complex
Light, leave-in conditioning mousse adds body and volume making hair firmer and stronger.

DANDRUFF

Clarifying Cleanser Contains Climbazole, a proven anti-dandruff ingredient that has an antibacterial effect, to give long-lasting protection against new scales forming. Effective help for dry or greasy dandruff or scaly scalp conditions, it gently releases deposits whilst smoothing and protecting against dryness.

Clarifying Amino Complex
Soothing conditioner containing Octopyrox, an effective anti-dandruff ingredient that helps re-generate the scalp and reduce inflammation.

HAIR LOSS

Ultimate Volume Cleanser
Herbal acids strengthen hair from
the inside while volumisers give
body and vitality.

Nutritive Tonic Stimulates the
hair follicle to promote healthy hair
growth and vitalises and cools the
scalp.

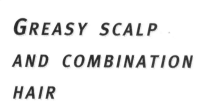

COLOURED HAIR

Colour Vitalising Cleanser
Natural extracts maintain colour
richness and help prevent colour
fade while silk proteins balance
moisture levels and give hair shine.

Colour Revitalising Complex
Brilliant leave-in care for coloured
hair adds shine and vibrance and
contains UV filters to protect
against fade.

DRY, SENSITIVE SCALP

Soothing Derma Cleanser
Extra-mild formulation that regu-
lates moisture, reduces inflammation, soothes the scalp and reduces
itching.

Soothing Derma Complex
Rich moisturiser that contains aloe
vera to soothe irritation and add
moisture to the scalp.

GREASY SCALP AND COMBINATION HAIR

Active Balancing Cleanser
Powerful anti-grease formulation
deep cleanses whilst regulating the
scalp's sebum production.

Active Balancing Complex
Intensive conditioner with Satinol, a
patented anti-grease ingredient that
prevents sebum distribution. A
volumiser lifts hair from the scalp to
give lightness and prevent grease
from spreading.

PERMED HAIR

Perm Energising Cleanser
Forms a protective cover around
each hair to give spring, elasticity
and volume to each curl.

Perm Energising Complex
Leave-in spray gives new elasticity
to permed hair, making curls last
longer by regulating the moisture
level and balancing the hair
structure.

*T*o maintain the benefits of a professional cleansing, conditioning and intensive treatment regime it is important to use styling products that are designed to maintain the reparative process.

Texturising Mousse Alcohol-free mousse gives springiness, volume and ultimate control.

Volumising Spray Conditioning blow-dry lotion for light to medium hold maintains the natural moisture level in hair whilst increasing bounce.

Designing Fluid Strong-hold, non-sticky styling lotion gives maximum manageability, especially for damaged hair.

Defining Gel Versatile, alchohol-free styling and finishing gel.

Contains mineral shine crystals to give hair superb, long-lasting shine with natural control and movement.

Controlling Spray Microfine spray gives natural hold and a silky shine with added protection against humidity.

Finishing Spray Strong-hold hairspray gives flexibility and volume without stickiness.

Wella System Professional Salon-size products are refillable and home-use bottles are stamped for ease of recycling.

Only available from Wella appointed salons worldwide.

WELLA

Wella Great Britain, Wella Road, Basingstoke, RG22 4AF, UK. Tel.: 01256 20202. Fax: 01256 471518.

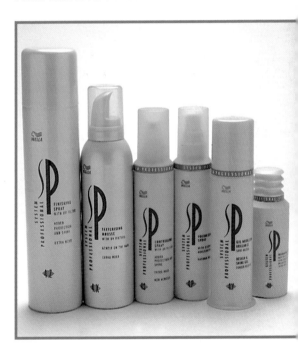

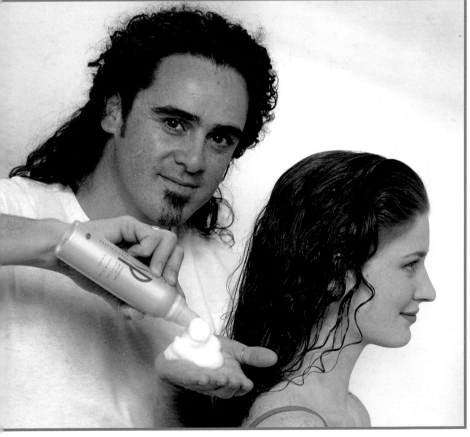

If you would like to learn more about dressing long hair, Patrick Cameron's 'Long Awaited' step-by-step educational videos will inspire and excite you.

Volume 1 features six long hair designs from Patrick's European collection.
Running time 45 minutes.
In **Volume 2**, Patrick presents a magical mix of twists and weaves and shares his secrets to instant elegance.
Running time 60 minutes.

Both videos are available by mail order from:
Patrick Cameron Hair International, PO Box 124, Chester, CH1 6ZF, UK.
Prices on application. Tel.: 0151 650 1403. Fax: 0151 650 1990.

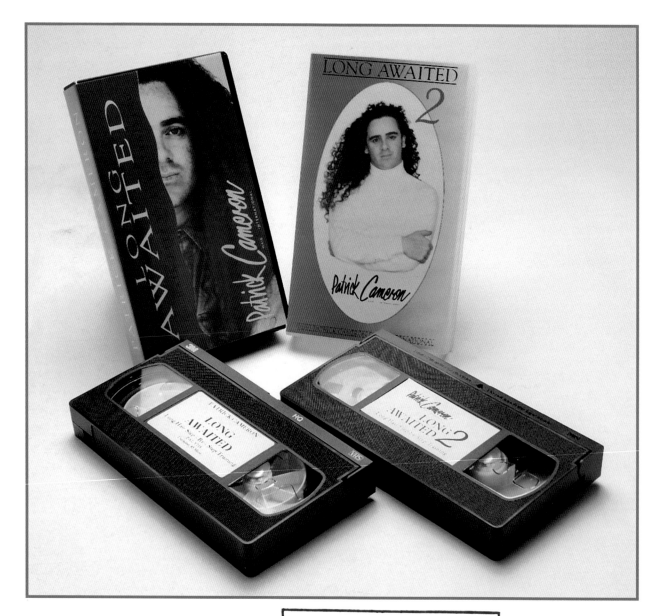

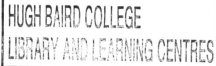